THE WASHINGTON MANUAL™

Allergy, Asthma, and Immunology

Subspecialty Consult

Second Edition

Editors

Shirley Joo, MD
Assistant Professor of Medicine
Division of Allergy and Immunology
Department of Internal Medicine
Washington University School of
    Medicine
St. Louis, Missouri

Andrew L. Kau, MD, PhD
Instructor in Medicine
Division of Allergy and Immunology
Department of Internal Medicine
Washington University School of
    Medicine
St. Louis, Missouri

Series Editors

Thomas M. De Fer, MD
*Associate Professor of Internal
    Medicine*
Washington University School of
    Medicine
St. Louis, Missouri

Katherine E. Henderson, MD
Assistant Professor of Clinical Medicine
Department of Medicine
Division of Medical Education
Washington University School of
    Medicine
Barnes-Jewish Hospital
St. Louis, Missouri

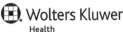 Wolters Kluwer | Lippincott Williams & Wilkins
Health
Philadelphia · Baltimore · New York · London
Buenos Aires · Hong Kong · Sydney · Tokyo

Senior Acquisitions Editor: Sonya Seigafuse
Senior Product Manager: Kerry Barrett
Vendor Manager: Bridgett Dougherty
Senior Marketing Manager: Kimberly Schonberger
Editorial Coordinator: Katie Sharp
Senior Manufacturing Manager: Ben Rivera
Design Coordinator: Holly McLaughlin
Production Service: Aptara, Inc.

Library of Congress Cataloging-in-Publication Data
The Washington manual™ allergy, asthma, and immunology subspecialty
consult. – 2nd ed. / edited by Shirley Joo and Andrew L. Kau.
    p. ; cm. – (Washington manual subspecialty consult series)
  Allergy, asthma, and immunology subspecialty consult
  Includes bibliographical references and index.
  ISBN 978-1-4511-1367-9 (alk. paper) – ISBN 1-4511-1367-6 (alk. paper)
  I. Joo, Shirley. II. Kau, Andrew L. III. Washington University (Saint
Louis, Mo.). Dept. of Medicine. IV. Title: Allergy, asthma, and immunology subspecialty consult.
V. Series: Washington manual subspecialty consult series.
  [DNLM: 1. Hypersensitivity–diagnosis–Handbooks.
2. Hypersensitivity–therapy–Handbooks. WD 300]
  616.97′5–dc23

                                                                    2012011793

                                                            10 9 8 7 6 5 4 3 2

Contributing Authors

Gregg J. Berdy, MD
*Assistant Professor of Clinical
   Ophthalmology and Visual Sciences*
Department of Ophthalmology and
   Visual Sciences
Washington University School of Medicine
St. Louis, Missouri

Susan S. Berdy, MD
Assistant Professor of Clinical Medicine
Department of Internal Medicine
Washington University School of Medicine
St. Louis, Missouri

Ashley Emmert, MD
Fellow in Allergy Immunology
Division of Allergy and Immunology
Department of Internal Medicine
Washington University School of Medicine
St. Louis, Missouri

Olajumoke O. Fadugba, MD
Senior Assistant Resident
Department of Internal Medicine
Washington University School of Medicine
St. Louis, Missouri

Bob Geng, MD
Senior Assistant Resident
Department of Internal Medicine
Washington University School of Medicine
St. Louis, Missouri

Seth M. Hollander, MD
Fellow in Allergy Immunology
Division of Allergy and Immunology
Department of Internal Medicine
Washington University School of Medicine
St. Louis, Missouri

Eric Karlin, MD
Senior Assistant Resident
Department of Internal Medicine
Washington University School of Medicine
St. Louis, Missouri

Andrew L. Kau, MD, PhD
Instructor in Medicine
Division of Allergy and Immunology
Department of Internal Medicine
Washington University School of Medicine
St. Louis, Missouri

Sydney Leibel, MD
Instructor in Pediatrics
Division of Pediatric Allergy, Immunology
   and Pulmonary Medicine
Department of Pediatrics
Washington University School of Medicine
St. Louis, Missouri

Seema Mahale, MD
Senior Assistant Resident
Department of Internal Medicine
Washington University School of Medicine
St. Louis, Missouri

K. Lindsey B. McMullan, MD
Fellow in Allergy Immunology
Division of Allergy and Immunology
Department of Internal Medicine
Washington University School of Medicine
St. Louis, Missouri

Natalie Miller, MD
Fellow in Allergy/Immunology
Division of Pediatric Allergy, Immunology,
   and Pulmonary Medicine
Department of Pediatrics
Washington University School of Medicine
St. Louis, Missouri

Sarena Sawlani, MD
Fellow in Allergy/Immunology
Division of Allergy and Immunology
Department of Internal Medicine
Washington University School of Medicine
St. Louis, Missouri

James A. Tarbox, MD
Fellow in Allergy/Immunology
Division of Allergy and Immunology
Department of Internal Medicine
Washington University School of Medicine
St. Louis, Missouri

Amanda Trott, MD
Fellow in Allergy/Immunology
Division of Pediatric Allergy, Immunology,
    and Pulmonary Medicine
Department of Pediatrics
Washington University School of Medicine
St. Louis, Missouri

Jennifer M. Welch, MD
Fellow in Allergy/Immunology
Division of Allergy and Immunology
Department of Internal Medicine
Washington University School of Medicine
St. Louis, Missouri

Chairman's Note

I t is a pleasure to present the new edition of *The Washington Manual*™ Subspecialty Consult Series: *Allergy, Asthma, and Immunology Subspecialty Consult*. This pocket-size book continues to be a primary reference for medical students, interns, residents, and other practitioners who need ready access to practical clinical information to diagnose and treat patients with a wide variety of disorders. Medical knowledge continues to increase at an astounding rate, which creates a challenge for physicians to keep up with the biomedical discoveries, genetic and genomic information, and novel therapeutics that can positively impact patient outcomes. The *Washington Manual*™ Subspecialty Consult Series addresses this challenge by concisely and practically providing current scientific information for clinicians to aid them in the diagnosis, investigation, and treatment of common medical conditions.

I want to personally thank the authors, who include house officers, fellows, and attendings at Washington University School of Medicine and Barnes Jewish Hospital. Their commitment to patient care and education is unsurpassed, and their efforts and skill in compiling this manual are evident in the quality of the final product. In particular, I would like to acknowledge our editors, Drs. Andrew L. Kau and Shirley Joo, and the series editors, Drs. Tom De Fer and Katherine Henderson, who have worked tirelessly to produce another outstanding edition of this manual. I would also like to thank Dr. Melvin Blanchard, Chief of the Division of Medical Education in the Department at of Medicine at Washington University School of Medicine, for his advice and guidance. I believe this edition of the *Allergy, Asthma, and Immunology Subspecialty Consult* will meet its desired goal of providing practical knowledge that can be directly applied at the bedside and in outpatient settings to improve patient care.

Victoria J. Fraser, MD
Dr. J. William Campbell Professor
Interim Chairman of Medicine
Co-Director of the Infectious Disease Division
Washington University School of Medicine

Preface

This is the second edition of the *Allergy, Asthma, and Immunology Subspecialty Consult*, which incorporates many significant updates to the prior edition, reflecting current clinical practices and understanding of allergic and immunologic diseases. Since its inception nearly 70 years ago, the *Washington Manual*™ has been written with the goal of conveying relevant and up-to-date medical information in a clear and concise manner. Like the first edition, this edition of the *Allergy, Asthma, and Immunology Subspecialty Consult* was written in the tradition of the *Washington Manual*™, with the intent of informing the reader about current practice in allergy and immunology.

The content of this second edition was written by the residents, fellows, and staff of the Washington University Department of Medicine. We have written this manual as a reference tool for interested interns, residents, medical students, and primary care physicians. Fellows-in-training and other health care professionals will also find it to be a succinct but thorough reference tool.

We would like to acknowledge our appreciation for the excellent work of the authors of the first edition of the *Allergy, Asthma, and Immunology Subspecialty Consult*, especially the editors, Dr. Barbara C. Jost, Dr. Elizabeth Friedman, Dr. Khaled M. Abdel-Hamid, Dr. Alpa L. Jani, and Dr. Tammy L. Lin. Finally, we would like to thank our excellent mentors, including Dr. H. James Wedner, Dr. Anthony Kulczycki, Dr. Philip E. Korenblat, Dr. Jeffrey Tillinghast, Dr. Rand Dankner, and Dr. Jacqueline Reiss.

—A.L.K.
—S.J.

Contents

Contributing Authors iii

Chairman's Note v

Preface vi

1 Approach to the Allergic Patient 1
Seth M. Hollander

2 Basic Immunology Underlying Allergic Reactions and Inflammation 4
Jennifer M. Welch and Andrew L. Kau

3 Allergic Rhinitis and Sinusitis 8
K. Lindsey B. McMullan

4 Asthma 23
Natalie Miller and Sarena Sawlani

5 Occupational Asthma 37
Seema Mahale

6 Hypersensitivity Pneumonitis 44
Olajumoke O. Fadugba

7 Pulmonary Function Tests 51
Ashley Emmert

8 *In Vivo* and *In Vitro* Diagnostic Tests of Allergy 59
Seth M. Hollander

9 Urticaria and Angioedema 68
James A. Tarbox

10 Atopic Dermatitis 77
Amanda Trott

11 Allergic Contact Dermatitis 85
Olajumoke O. Fadugba

12 Ocular Allergic Disease **89**
Gregg J. Berdy and Susan S. Berdy

13 Anaphylaxis **96**
Sydney Leibel

14 Drug Allergy and Desensitization **103**
Jennifer M. Welch

15 Insect Allergy **116**
K. Lindsey B. McMullan

16 Food Allergy and Other Adverse Food Reactions **125**
Amanda Trott

17 Latex Hypersensitivity **135**
Eric Karlin

18 Conditions Associated with Eosinophilia **140**
Bob Geng

19 Mastocytosis **154**
Bob Geng

20 Primary Immunodeficiency Diseases **160**
Sydney Leibel

21 Allergen Immunotherapy **173**
James A. Tarbox

Appendixes
A. Common Medications Used in Allergy and Immunology **181**
B. Lab Values for Selected Tests in Immunology **189**
C. Sample Schedule for Perennial Aqueous Immunotherapy **194**

Index **195**

Approach to the Allergic Patient

Seth M. Hollander

GENERAL PRINCIPLES

Definition

- The term *allergy* is credited to the pediatrician Clemons von Pirquet who in 1906 used it to describe an "altered biologic reactivity." This was not only in reference to immunity against disease but also to hypersensitivity leading to tissue damage.[1]
- The modern definition of allergy is an overreaction or abnormal response of the immune system to innocuous substances.[1]

DIAGNOSIS

Clinical Presentation

History
- As with most disorders in medicine, the most important component in diagnosing allergic disorders is taking a thorough history.
- Identify the symptom location, character, and frequency, as well as the alleviating and exacerbating factors.
- Exacerbating or alleviating factors:
  - Seasonal variation of symptoms
  - Prior response to medications
  - Reactions to specific and nonspecific exposures
    - Pets.
    - Smoke, irritant fumes.
    - Perfume.
    - Change in temperature.
    - Food, medications, etc.

Environmental History
- Common relevant environmental exposures exacerbating symptoms may not be obvious to the patient.
- Typical questions that may help to identify relevant exposures include:
  - Location of home: Rural, urban, suburban.
  - Work exposures.
  - Hobbies, sports, etc.
  - Presence of water damage at home or work place or visible mold.
  - Presence of pets.
  - Age of mattress/bedding.
  - Age of carpeting at home.

Family History
- Allergic diseases have a strong hereditary link.
- A parental history of allergic rhinitis increases a 6-year old's odds of allergic rhinitis by 1.84 (1.16–2.94).[2]
- A parental history of asthma increases a 6-year old's odds of asthma by 2.72 (1.19–6.18).[2]
- A maternal history of eczema or atopy increases a 6-month old's risk of eczema by 1.58 (1.01–2.47) and 1.99 (1.43–2.78), respectively.[3]

Food Allergy History
- While allergies to food are thought to be much more common in children, they are also seen in adults in comparable numbers.[4]
- Food allergies are often implicated, (with a prevalence of 3–35%),[4] more often than they are proven to be true (actual prevalence rate of 1–10.8% after oral food challenge[4,5]). A thorough history can lead to appropriate testing, which may further help to confirm or exclude suspected foods.

Physical Examination
General Appearance
- Nasal congestion can lead to a "nasal" or "adenoidal" sounding voice as well as mouth breathing.
- Nasal tissue edema may lead to compression of the draining veins under the eyes. This can manifest as dark regions under the eyes often called "**allergic shiners.**"
- Infraorbital folds or **Dennie–Morgan lines** may be present.
- Patients may be observed to rub upward across their nose with the palm of the hand. This is known as the "**allergic salute**" and may cause a transverse line across the lower portion of the nose or nasal crease.

Head and Neck
- Eyes are commonly noted to have conjunctival injection and watering due to allergic disease.
- Common allergic features of the nose include swollen, edematous turbinates that are pale blue in color.
- Presence of nasal polyps which often appear like clear whitish sacs hanging from the underside of a turbinate.
- Close examination of nasal septum to assess presence of perforations or deviations.
- Tympanic membranes may be dull with the presence of effusion behind them.
- **Flexible rhinoscopy** is helpful in looking closer at the turbinate anatomy and vocal cords to assess for the presence of nasal polyps, sinusitis, or vocal cord dysfunction.

Pulmonary
- A thorough lung exam is required, including auscultation of all lung fields, to listen for any evidence of wheezing or an increased expiratory phase.
- If wheezing cannot be heard during a standard exam, a forced expiratory maneuver may be helpful.

Skin
- **Urticaria,** or hives, is a maculopapular erythematous eruption in the cutaneous tissues. These can range from pinpoint size to multiple inches in diameter and are typically pruritic and blanch with pressure.

- **Angioedema** is edema of the subcutaneous tissue; nonpruritic and often painful.
- **Dermatographism** is the tendency to form a wheal and flair response when firm pressure is applied to the skin.
- **Atopic dermatitis** is associated with allergic disease. This presents as dry, scaly, pruritic patches occurring at typical locations depending on the age of the patient.

Diagnostic Testing

As with all testing, the results must be interpreted with appropriate clinical context as to distinguish between sensitization and symptomatic allergy.

Skin Testing

- This is the most rapid and specific method to test for allergic sensitivity.
- Two methods are commonly used, and both are discussed in Chapter 8:
  - Epicutaneous testing.
  - Intradermal testing.

In Vitro Tests

- *In vitro* testing (radioallergosorbent test [RAST] and ImmunoCAP) is designed to screen for the presence of allergen-specific immunoglobulin E (IgE) in the patient's serum.
- These methods have lower sensitivity and specificity compared to epicutaneous skin testing but are helpful in instances where skin testing cannot be performed.

Pulmonary Testing

- When a history of breathing difficulties, wheezing, or coughing is reported, pulmonary function tests are often needed to evaluate for asthma.
- Occasionally a plain chest radiograph is helpful.
- When standard pulmonary function tests are normal, but there is still a high suspicion for asthma, modifications may be needed as follows:
  - Exercise spirometry.
  - Bronchoprovocation challenge (i.e., methacholine or mannitol).

REFERENCES

1. Jamieson M. Imagining 'reactivity': allergy within the history of immunology. *Stud Hist Philos Biol Biomed Sci.* 2010;41:356–366.
2. Alford SH, Zoratti E, Peterson E, et al. Parental history of atopic disease: disease pattern and risk of pediatric atopy in offspring. *J Allergy Clin Immunol.* 2004;114:1046–1050.
3. Moore MM, Rifas-Shiman SL, Rich-Edwards JW, et al. Perinatal predictors of atopic dermatitis occurring in the first six months of life. *Pediatrics.* 2004;113:468–474.
4. Rona RR, Keil T, Summers C, et al. The prevalence of food allergy: a meta-analysis. *J Allergy Clin Immunol.* 2007;120:638–646.
5. Lieberman JA, Sicherer SH. Diagnosis of food allergy: epicutaneous skin tests, in vitro tests, and oral food challenge. *Curr Allergy Asthma Rep.* 2011;11:8–64.

Basic Immunology Underlying Allergic Reactions and Inflammation

2

Jennifer M. Welch and Andrew L. Kau

GENERAL PRINCIPLES

Definitions

- The immune system is responsible for protecting us from bacterial, viral, fungal, and helminthic pathogens. At the same time, the immune system must remain tolerant to self-derived antigens, antigens present on commensal organisms, proteins in food, and antigens present in the environment.
  - **Autoimmunity** results when there is loss of immunologic tolerance to "self"-antigens.
  - **Allergy** is the result of loss of tolerance to environmental or food antigens (also called allergens).
  - **Immunodeficiency** describes the lack of appropriate immune response to a pathogen that results in recurrent infection.
- Components of the immune system include the innate and adaptive systems.

Innate Immune System

- The innate immune system comprises lymphoid-derived cells (e.g., neutrophils, macrophages, dendritic cells, eosinophils, etc.), non-lymphoid tissues (e.g., epithelial cells), and proteins capable of pathogen recognition.
- Innate immune cells are able to identify pathogens through **pattern recognition receptors** (PRR) that distinguish conserved features of pathogens, termed **pathogen-associated molecular patterns** (PAMP).

Adaptive Immune System

- **Cellular immunity, or cell-mediated immunity,** consists of the response mediated by T cells.
- Types of **CD4+ T cells** are classified by the type of cytokines that they express:
  - T_H1 cells express cytokines such as interferon-γ and help respond to bacteria, viruses, mycobacteria, and some parasites.
  - T_H2 cells express cytokines like interleukin (IL)-4, IL-5, IL-13 and protect from parasitic infections. Inappropriate activation of the T_H2 response is associated with allergy.
  - Tregs (or regulatory T cells) are a subset of T cells that mediate tolerance to both self-antigens and exogenous antigens. They express immunoregulatory cytokines such as transforming growth factor (TGF)-β.
- **Humoral immunity** is mediated by antibodies produced by B cells.
  - Immunoglobulin G (IgG) is present primarily in the serum and helps protect from viral and bacterial pathogens.
  - IgA is produced primarily on mucosal surfaces, protects against pathogens on the mucosal surface, and helps maintain homeostasis with colonizing microbes.
  - IgE is thought to protect from parasitic infections and is responsible for allergic reactions.

TABLE 2-1	HYPERSENSITIVITY REACTIONS	
Type	Mechanism	Examples
I	IgE-mediated mast cell degranulation and activation	Allergic rhinitis, anaphylaxis, acute urticaria, atopic dermatitis, food allergy, insect sting allergy, allergic asthma
II	IgG or IgM binds antigen on cell surface, causing phagocytosis or complement-mediated cellular destruction	Autoimmune or drug-induced hemolytic anemia, Rh incompatibility, Goodpasture's disease
III	Immune complex–mediated disease	Serum sickness, hypersensitivity pneumonitis, systemic lupus erythematosus, vasculitis
IV	Delayed-type hypersensitivity (T-cell mediated)	Tuberculin reaction, allograft rejection, graft-vs-host disease, contact dermatitis

IgE, immunoglobulin E; IgG, immunoglobulin G; IgM, immunoglobulin M.

Classification

Gell–Coombs provides a classification for immune-mediated hypersensitivity reactions and is divided into four types that are shown in Table 2-1.

Etiology

- Allergy develops when B cells are stimulated to produce IgE antibody to an environmental or food antigen.
- The **hygiene hypothesis** was formulated to help explain the increase of allergic disease in developed countries over the past few decades. It postulates that reduced exposure to infections in early childhood due to improved living standards, hygiene, and smaller family size results in less T_H1 stimulation and thus an increase in T_H2-mediated diseases.
- Children living in rural areas with heavy exposure to animals have a lower prevalence of allergy and asthma compared to children living in the same area without exposure to animals.[1]
- **Antigens** that mediate allergic reactions (also called allergens) comprise a wide variety of molecules, including chemicals and proteins commonly encountered in a person's environment. Examples include dust mite, pollen, and animal dander. Some chemicals are able to elicit an immune response by binding to self-proteins creating a hapten–carrier conjugate. This is seen in penicillin allergy.
- **IgE** is a 190 kD immunoglobulin found in minute amounts in the serum. It circulates as a bivalent antibody, and in pathologic conditions, such as parasitic infection or severe atopy, these levels can rise in the serum. IgE is synthesized by B cells that are activated and differentiated into plasma cells that secrete IgE.
  - Activation of B cells to make IgE requires IL-4 or IL-13 as a helper signal that is secreted by T_H2 helper CD4+ cells.
  - Once secreted, IgE binds to Fc receptors on tissue mast cells to sensitize these cells to allergens.

○ There are two main types of **IgE receptors**, a high-affinity Fc receptor called FcεRI and a low-affinity Fc receptor called FcεRII. The high-affinity receptor is located on mast cells, basophils, dendritic cells, eosinophils, and Langerhans cells.
  ▪ The **high-affinity FcεRI receptor** is composed of α-chain that binds to the Fc portion of IgE, a β-chain and two γ-chains that are involved with intracellular signaling. Eosinophils do not contain the β-chain.
  ▪ The presence of IgE increases FcεRI expression on the surface of mast cells. Individuals with higher IgE levels need a smaller trigger for mast cell activation.
• The **allergic response** is composed of two phases: Immediate and late phase.
  ○ The **immediate response** occurs when antigen binds to mast cell–associated IgE (which is bound to the surface of the mast cell by its high-affinity receptor, FcεR1). This causes cross-linking of IgE and stimulates mast cell to release its preformed granules. This reaction can appear within 5–10 minutes after the administration of antigen and usually subsides in an hour. The wheal-and-flare response seen during allergy skin testing (see Chapter 8) is an example of an immediate allergic response.
  ○ The **late-phase reaction** is mediated by cytokines and lipid mediators produced by mast cells along with neutrophils, eosinophils, basophils, and T_H2 T cells recruited to the site. The late-phase reaction occurs 2–4 hours after the immediate response, and the inflammation is maximal by 24 hours before it subsides. Late-phase allergic inflammation can be reduced with corticosteroids but not antihistamines.
• **Mast cells** arise from CD34+ bone marrow progenitors and migrate as immature cells to peripheral tissue where they mature near blood vessels, nerves, and beneath epithelia. Mast cells vary in shape and have round nuclei with cytoplasmic granules containing acidic proteoglycans that bind to basic dyes.
  ○ Activated mast cells are a key component to allergic reactions. They secrete various mediators that are either stored pre-formed in granules or synthesized upon activation.
  ○ **Pre-formed granules** consist of biogenic amines (histamine), neutral proteases (tryptase, chymase, carboxypeptidase), acid hydrolases, proteoglycans (heparin, chondroitin sulfate), and tumor necrosis factor (TNF)-α. These are released within minutes of cross-linking of surface-bound IgE.
  ○ **Histamine** acts upon release on the four different histamine receptors. Its actions are short lived, because it is rapidly removed from the extracellular space.
    ▪ Through the H_1 receptor, histamine causes smooth muscle contraction (bronchospasm), pruritus, vasodilation, and vasopermeability. This creates the wheal-and-flare response on the skin.
    ▪ The H_2 receptor is responsible for gastric acid secretion and increased mucus production in the airways.
    ▪ The H_3 receptor is found in the nervous system and controls the release of histamine and other neurotransmitters.
    ▪ The H_4 receptor aids in chemotaxis of mast cells.
  ○ **Tryptase is found only in mast cells and is a marker of mast cell activation.** Tryptase cleaves fibrinogen and activates collagenase causing tissue damage. Tryptase is found in two forms, α-tryptase and β-tryptase.
    ▪ α-Tryptase is constitutively secreted. Levels are elevated in the disease mastocytosis.
    ▪ β-Tryptase is released upon mast cell degranulation. It is stabilized by heparin. Blood level peak 30 minutes after anaphylactic reaction but may remain above baseline level for 6–12 hours after inciting event.
  ○ **Synthesized mediators** are made by mast cells minutes to hours after activation and include arachidonic acid metabolites and cytokines.

○ Lipid metabolites are created from arachidonic acid via the cyclooxygenase or lipoxygenase pathways and are mediators in allergic reactions.

- **Prostaglandin D$_2$** (PGD$_2$) is synthesized through the cyclooxygenase pathway. PGD$_2$ acts on smooth muscle cells to mediate vasodilatation and bronchoconstriction. It also promotes neutrophil chemotaxis.
- **Leukotrienes** are created via the lipoxygenase pathways. Leukotriene C$_4$ (LTC$_4$) is made by mucosal mast cells and is degraded to LTD$_4$ and LTE$_4$. These are important mediators of asthmatic bronchoconstriction. In addition, they also increase vascular permeability and mucus secretion.
- **Platelet-activating factor** (PAF) causes bronchoconstriction, vascular permeability, relaxes vascular smooth muscle, and can activate leukocytes. PAF has a short half life as it is rapidly destroyed. It received its name as it causes rabbit platelet aggregation.

○ **Mast cell synthesized cytokines** that contribute to allergic inflammation include the following:

- IL-3 induces mast cell proliferation.
- IL-4 and IL-13 promote IgE isotype switching and mucus secretion.
- IL-5 activates and induces eosinophil proliferation.
- IL-6 promotes B-cell differentiation.
- TNF-α activates endothelial expression of adhesion molecules that aid in leukocyte recruitment.

○ Mast cells can be stimulated to release their mediators by:

- Allergens binding to surface IgE on mast cells causing cross-linking. Cross-linking describes the process of simultaneous engagement of multiple IgE Fc receptors necessary for signaling.
- Antibody binding to IgE or FcεR1 receptor causing cross-linking.
- Histamine releasing factors that include chemokines such as macrophage inflammatory protein (MIP)-1, complement factors C3a and C5a, and neuropeptides like substance P.
- Drugs (morphine, codeine) and IV contrast dye.
- Physical stimuli such as pressure, heat, cold, and sunlight.

• **Basophils** are a blood granulocyte with a similar function and structure to mast cells.

○ Their name is derived from the ability of their granules to bind to basic dye. Basophils can synthesize many of the same mediators as mast cells.

○ Basophils also express FcεR1 receptor and can be activated by antigen binding to IgE.

○ Basophils make up less than 1% of blood leukocytes. They are normally not present in tissue, but may be recruited to sites of inflammation.

• **Eosinophils** are a blood granulocyte that is commonly involved in allergic diseases.

○ Eosinophil maturation is promoted by granulocyte macrophage colony-stimulating factor (GM-CSF), IL-3, and IL-5. They are normally seen in peripheral tissue and are recruited to sites of inflammation mainly in the late-phase reaction.

○ Their granules contain basic proteins that bind to acidic dye. Eosinophils have receptors for IgG, IgA, and IgE. Once activated, eosinophils produce major basic protein, eosinophil cationic protein, and eosinophil peroxidase, which are toxic to bacteria, helminths, and normal tissue. They can also release lipid mediators that aid in the allergic response.

REFERENCE

1. von Mutius E. Influences in allergy: epidemiology and the environment. *J Allergy Clin Immunol.* 2004;113:373–379.

Allergic Rhinitis and Sinusitis

3

K. Lindsey B. McMullan

RHINITIS

GENERAL PRINCIPLES

- One of the most common chronic diseases, allergic rhinitis (AR) is characterized by rhinorrhea, nasal congestion, postnasal drainage, nasopharyngeal itching, and sneezing.
- AR symptoms are caused by environmental allergens.
- The prevalence of AR is increasing.
- Rhinitis includes AR, nonallergic rhinitis (NAR), and nonallergic rhinitis with eosinophilia syndrome (NARES).

Definition

- AR is allergen-driven mucosal inflammation.
- AR must contain one or more of the following symptoms:[1]
  ○ Nasal congestion
  ○ Sneezing
  ○ Itching
  ○ Rhinorrhea
  ○ Postnasal drip
- For rhinitis to be classified as allergic, the patient must have **evidence of immunoglobulin E (IgE) sensitization to an allergen** by skin testing or radioallergosorbent test (RAST).
- Other associated symptoms include palatal pruritus, pruritus of the ear canals, ocular pruritus and watering, and some patients have anosmia or reduced sense of smell.
- **Nonallergic rhinitis** (NAR) is not mediated by IgE.
  ○ There is nasal mucosal inflammation.
  ○ Symptoms are similar to AR usually without itching.
  ○ No sensitization to allergens is demonstrated.
- **NARES** is NAR with eosinophilia syndrome.
  ○ Symptoms are very similar or identical to AR.
  ○ There is no IgE sensitization to allergen.
  ○ Large numbers of eosinophils are present on nasal smear (may be >20%).
  ○ Patients tend to be middle-aged and often have paroxysmal exacerbations.
  ○ Patients are at increased risk for obstructive sleep apnea.[1]

Classification

- **Allergic rhinitis** can be classified into seasonal, perennial, and episodic.
  ○ **Seasonal AR:** Patients have signs and symptoms of AR occurring in only one or more seasons, but not year round. They are sensitized to seasonal allergens such as trees, grasses, or weeds.

- ○ **Perennial AR:** Patients have signs and symptoms of AR throughout the year, though they may also have seasonal exacerbations if they are sensitized to seasonal allergens.
  - Allergens typically include dust mites, molds, pet dander, or insects.
  - Symptoms must be present >2 hours/day, >9 months out of the year.
  - ○ **Episodic AR:** Patients have signs and symptoms of AR to allergens they are sensitized to, but which are not present regularly in their environment. An example would be a patient who has symptoms when visiting a friend who has a cat, but the patient does not come into daily contact with the cat.[1]
- **Mixed rhinitis:** Patients have a combination of AR and NAR.

Epidemiology

- AR affects between 10 and 30% of all adults.[1]
- Mixed rhinitis affects 44–87% of patients with rhinitis.[1,2]
- In 2002, the financial burden in the US (direct and indirect costs) was estimated at $11.58 billion.[1]
- Prevalence ranges from 3 to 19%.
- 80% of AR develops before age 20.
- Equal male and female distribution among adults.
- Adults have a higher prevalence of perennial AR and children have a higher prevalence of seasonal AR.

Etiology

- **Allergens:** Sensitization to aeroallergens may occur even in the first 2 years of life.[1]
- **Anatomic causes** of rhinitis include septal deviation, foreign bodies, adenoid hypertrophy, choanal atresia, and tumors.

Pathophysiology

- AR is caused by specific **IgE-mediated** reaction to environmental allergens.
- Mast cells and basophils located on the superficial mucosa of the respiratory tract have specific IgE bound to its cell membrane. When allergens bind and cross-link the IgE, cellular degranulation occurs.
  - ○ Mast cells degranulate and cause release of pre-formed mediators and newly synthesized mediators that cause the allergic reaction.[2]
  - ○ Preformed mediators include histamine, tryptase, chymase, kininogenase, heparin, and other enzymes.
  - ○ Newly formed mediators include prostaglandins, leukotriene (LT) C4, LTD4, and LTE4.
- Nasal congestion is typically a late-phase response.
- Eosinophils release mediators causing tissue damage in the late phase response.[1]
- **Priming** occurs with prolonged allergen exposure resulting in repeated late-phase responses even with very small exposures—inflammatory mediators continue to be released and symptom resolution may lag behind the decrease in pollen.[1]
- NAR causes include hormonal, vasomotor, and medication-induced.

Risk Factors

- Family history of atopy.
- Serum IgE >100 IU/mL before age 6.
- Higher socioeconomic status.
- Presence of a positive skin prick test.[1]

- First-born children are more likely to have AR.
- Environmental risk factors include smoke exposure and allergen exposure in infancy.

DIAGNOSIS

Clinical Presentation

- Patients typically present with sneezing, rhinorrhea, postnasal drip, nasal itching, and congestion.[1]
- Other symptoms include itching of palate, conjunctiva, throat, Eustachian tubes, and middle ear.
- Ear fullness and popping, as well as pressure over cheeks and forehead may be reported.
- Occasionally, chronic cough may be the presenting symptom.
- Often patients can associate the onset of symptoms to a particular trigger.
- **Common comorbidities** include:[1]
  - Asthma.
  - Obstructive sleep apnea.
  - Nasal obstruction from severe nasal septal deviation.
  - Inferior turbinate hypertrophy.
  - Adenoidal hypertrophy.
  - Refractory sinusitis.
  - Allergic conjunctivitis.

History

- History is the **most important step** in diagnosis.
- Important elements of the history:
  - Frequency of symptoms.
  - Severity of symptoms (both past and present).
  - Relationship to past symptoms.
  - Length of time symptoms appear after triggers.
- **Triggers** may be multiple.
- Assess whether the symptoms occur at home and/or work on vacation.
- Assessment of **home environmental conditions** should include:
  - Water damage or mold.
  - Pets.
  - Carpet.
  - Age of pillow and mattress, type of fillers.
  - What other irritants are nearby (e.g., farms, woods, and vacant lots)?
  - Are heat and air conditioning central?
  - Use of fireplace or humidifiers.
  - Are symptoms exacerbated by dusting or vacuuming the house?
- **Medications** specifically inquire about:
  - Does the patient take aspirin, nonsteroidal anti-inflammatory drugs (NSAIDs), oral contraceptives, angiotensin-converting enzyme (ACE)-inhibitors, or β-blockers?
  - What are current and past medications used to treat AR?
- **Family history of atopic disease** should be determined.
- **Quality of life** should be assessed.
  - Ask about fatigue, learning and attention problems, and sleep disturbance.
  - Ask about time missed from work or school.
  - Effect on quality of life is often under-recognized and inadequately treated.[1]
- Rhinorrhea should be described as predominately clear. Persistent, colored rhinorrhea may indicate sinus disease.

- Time frame of exacerbations should be established.
  - ○ Are symptoms always worse on awakening?
  - ○ Are there particular seasons that are worse?
  - ○ Are symptoms completely gone during portions of the year?

Physical Examination
- A thorough examination of the head, eyes, ears, nose, and throat should be performed.
- Note if findings are unilateral or bilateral.
- Common findings in AR include:
  - ○ **Allergic salute** is a crease across the bridge of the nose and is a result of rubbing the nose.
  - ○ **Dennie's lines** are infraorbital creases.
  - ○ **Conjunctivitis** may be present in those with ocular symptoms.
  - ○ **Allergic shiners** are infraorbital hyperpigmentation secondary to nasal congestion.
  - ○ Turbinates are often edematous and pale. They may sometimes appear blue.
  - ○ **Cobblestoning** in the posterior oropharynx indicates post-nasal drainage.
  - ○ Ears should be evaluated for otitis or Eustachian tube dysfunction.
  - ○ It should be noted whether **septal deviation** or **nasal polyps** are present.
  - ○ Care should be taken to ensure there is no sinusitis (see below).
  - ○ Heart and lung examination should be performed. Note whether wheezing is heard on lung examination.
  - ○ The skin should be examined for signs of atopic dermatitis.
- If **septal perforation** is present, differential diagnosis includes:
  - ○ Inappropriate use of nasal medications.
  - ○ Adverse effects of other nasal medications.
  - ○ Intranasal narcotic abuse.
  - ○ Previous surgery.
  - ○ Systemic granulomatous disease.

Differential Diagnosis
- The differential diagnosis of rhinitis is presented in Table 3-1.

TABLE 3-1	DIFFERENTIAL DIAGNOSIS FOR RHINITIS
Allergic rhinitis	
Nonallergic rhinitis (NAR)	
Nonallergic rhinitis with eosinophilia syndrome (NARES)	
Vasomotor rhinitis	
Hormonal rhinitis	
Drug-induced rhinitis	
Atrophic rhinitis	
Gustatory rhinitis	
Infectious rhinitis	
Sinusitis	
Rhinitis medicamentosa	
Cystic fibrosis	
Ciliary dysfunction	
Cerebrospinal fluid rhinorrhea	
Anatomical abnormalities	
Nasal tumors	
Nasal polyps	
Foreign bodies	

- **Vasomotor rhinitis:**
  - This is a type of NAR in which excessive vasomotor activity leads to chronic nasal congestion.
  - The mechanism is not completely known.
  - Etiologies include **odors, alcohol, spicy foods, emotions, temperature change, and bright lights.**
- **Drug-induced rhinitis:**
  - Common offenders include ACE-inhibitors, β-blockers, ASA, NSAIDs, oral contraceptives, phosphodiesterase-5-selective inhibitors, α-receptor antagonists, and cocaine.
- **Hormonal rhinitis:**
  - A type of NAR in which hormone altering events induce nasal obstruction and hypersecretion.
  - Events include **hypothyroidism, oral contraceptive use, and pregnancy.**
  - For pregnant women, symptoms usually appear during the second trimester but disappear after delivery.
- **Rhinitis medicamentosa:**
  - Occurs from prolonged use of **intranasal decongestants.**
  - Rebound congestion occurs and later nasal hypertrophy. This appears as beefy, red mucosa.
  - Rhinitis medicamentosa will resolve on discontinuation of the agent.
- **Nasal polyps** are outgrowths from the nasal passages.
  - Polyps typically start at the lateral wall and appear smooth, round, pale, and gelatinous.
  - Growth likely occurs from eosinophil-associated growth factors found in the eosinophils and immunoglobulins they contain.
  - The possibility of cystic fibrosis should be entertained if nasal polyps are found in children.
- **Anatomic abnormalities** should be considered, particularly in difficult-to-treat rhinitis.
- If **cerebrospinal fluid (CSF) rhinorrhea** is suspected, evaluate with β-transferrin in nasal secretions.[1]

Diagnostic Testing

- **Skin testing** and **RAST testing** are used to determine allergen sensitization. These are discussed in detail in Chapter 8.
- Purposes of serum IgE testing are three-fold: To provide evidence of allergic basis, to confirm suspected allergens, and to determine suspected sensitivity for avoidance measures and/or immunotherapy.[1]
- Epicutaneous skin testing is preferred.
- Testing to local trees, weeds, and grasses is usually performed. Testing is also usually performed to molds and perennial allergens.

Laboratories

- **RAST testing** is usually used only if skin testing is unable to be performed.
- The average sensitivity of serum-specific IgE assays is only 70–75%.[1]
- Reasons for skin testing might be contraindicated include use of antihistamines, extensive skin disease, and uncooperative patients who are not able to sit still for 15–20 minutes.
- Serum IgE and IgG subclasses **are not** used as diagnostic tools for AR.

Imaging
If anatomic abnormality or chronic sinusitis is suspected, a CT scan may be helpful.

Diagnostic Procedures
- **Rhinoscopy** may be used to:
  - Assess nasal passage structure.
  - Evaluate for nasal polyps and sinusitis.
  - Evaluate vocal chords.
- **Nasal provocation testing** is rarely performed and is used primarily for research purposes to confirm sensitivity to allergen.[1]

TREATMENT

- When treatment with one class fails despite compliance, substitution of another class should be considered.
- If AR is mild, single-agent therapy or combination therapy may be used in addition to avoidance measures.
- For all intranasal preparations, patients should be instructed to spray medication **away from the septum** to avoid irritation and perforation.

Medications

First Line
- Intranasal steroids are the mainstay of therapy.
  - They are considered superior to all other medication choices for AR because they help prevent both early and late-phase response.
  - Steroids for intranasal use include beclomethasone, budesonide, flunisolide, fluticasone furoate, fluticasone propionate, mometasone, triamcinolone, and ciclesonide.
  - Typical adult dose is two sprays in each nostril daily.
  - Patients with seasonal AR should start intranasal steroids at least 1 week before the onset of pollen season.
  - May be used on an as needed basis but this is not as effective as daily use.
  - Systemic side effects are minimal.
  - Patients should be instructed on their proper use to prevent nasal septum trauma.
  - Nasal examination in patients on nasal steroids should evaluate for complications such as septal ulceration and perforation (rare).
  - Epistaxis may occur, and if frequent, discontinuation of the nasal steroid should be considered.
- Oral antihistamines are also commonly used.[3]
  - They reduce symptoms of rhinorrhea, nasal pruritus, sneezing, ocular pruritus, and tearing.
  - They are less effective at reducing nasal congestion.
  - Nonsedating second-generation antihistamines include loratadine, desloratadine, fexofenadine, cetirizine, and levocetirizine.
  - First-generation antihistamines are not generally used for AR secondary to their sedating properties. These include chlorpheniramine, diphenhydramine, doxepin, and hydroxyzine.
- Nasal antihistamines:
  - These may be as effective or superior to oral second-generation antihistamines.[1]
  - They are generally less effective than intranasal steroids.
  - Examples include azelastine and olopatadine.

Second Line

- **Montelukast** is approved for seasonal and perennial AR.
- **Intranasal cromolyn:**[1,3]
  - Inhibits mast cell degranulation.
  - Onset of action is 4–7 days.
  - Effective for episodic AR.
  - Must be used four times daily for maximal effect.
  - Has a good safety profile.
  - Is not as efficacious as nasal steroids or nasal antihistamines.
- **Intranasal anticholinergics (ipratropium):**[1,3]
  - Reduces rhinorrhea.
  - Not useful for nasal congestion.
  - Side effects include epistaxis and nasal dryness.
  - Use with caution in patients with glaucoma or prostate hypertrophy.
- **Nasal decongestants:**
  - Cause vasoconstriction and improve nasal edema, but no actual effect on the antigen-provoked nasal response.[1]
  - Should not be used as single agent.[3]
  - Continuous use should be limited to <5 days otherwise may lead to rhinitis medicamentosa.[3]
  - Examples are oxymetazoline and phenylephrine.
- **Oral decongestants:**
  - Are occasionally useful in selected patients.
  - Most products generally contain phenylephrine.
  - Chronic use of these agents is not recommended.[3]
- **Oral steroids:**
  - Are **rarely indicated** in AR secondary to systemic side effects.
  - For severe, intractable nasal symptoms or if nasal polyps are present, a 5- to 7-day course may be considered.
- **Immunotherapy** (see Chapter 21):
  - Immunotherapy may be used for treatment of perennial and seasonal rhinitis **when a specific allergen has been identified.**
  - Successful approximately 80% of the time.
  - Considered unsuccessful if the patient has no relief from symptoms after 1 year of maintenance therapy.
  - Current recommendations suggest 3–5 years of therapy.

Other Nonpharmacologic Therapies

- Environmental modification:
  - Dust mite avoidance:
    - Dust mite proof covers for mattresses and pillows are designed to help decrease the amount of dust mites and other allergens.
    - Vacuum with a HEPA filter.[1]
    - Wash linens in hot water.
    - Indoor humidity should be kept <50% to avoid growth of fungi and dust mites.[1]
    - Hard surface flooring is preferable
  - Avoid contact with pets. For cat allergen, the cat may be confined to a HEPA-filtered room.[1]

○ Pollen counts are highest on sunny, windy days with lower humidity.
  ■ Close windows and doors during pollen season.
  ■ Performing outdoor activity in the evening when pollen counts are lower.
○ Mold exposure should be avoided at home.
  ■ To eliminate fungi, sources of moisture should be eliminated initially.
  ■ Porous surfaces should be replaced.
○ Eliminate cockroaches (much easier said than done).
○ Wear a HEPA and pollen-proof face mask (e.g., N95) when allergens cannot be avoided.
• Nasal saline irrigations may help symptoms of chronic rhinitis.[1,4]

SPECIAL CONSIDERATIONS

Pregnancy
• Symptoms of AR increase in one-third of pregnant patients.[1]
• Both first- and second-generation antihistamines may be used. Cetirizine is a pregnancy class B medication.
• Oral decongestants should be avoided, particularly in the first trimester.
• Other medications that may be used include intranasal steroids (budesonide, beclomethasone, fluticasone propionate, class B), montelukast (class B), and sodium cromolyn (class B).
• Immunotherapy may be continued without dose escalation during pregnancy, but immunotherapy should not be initiated during pregnancy.

Elderly Patients
• Age-related changes such as cholinergic hyperactivity, anatomic changes, or concomitant medication use may affect rhinitis.
• Allergy is not a common cause of new onset rhinitis in persons >65 years.[2]
• Intranasal steroids and ipratropium may be used safely.
• If antihistamines are used, nonsedating agents should be chosen.[2]

COMPLICATIONS

• Medical complications of improperly or untreated AR include rhinosinusitis, otitis media, and rhinitis medicamentosa.[1]
• Psychological impact can include depression, anxiety, low self-esteem, and shyness.
• Septal irritation or perforation may occur as a complication of incorrect nasal steroid use.

REFERRAL

• There are **multiple indications** for referral to an allergist-immunologist (Table 3-2).
• Consultation with an allergist-immunologist has been demonstrated to improve outcomes such as compliance, quality of life, and patient satisfaction.[1]
• Patients that should be referred to an otolaryngologist for surgical management include:[1]
  ○ Nasal obstruction from severe nasal septal deviation (septoplasty is preferred over submucosal resection and has a high reported success rate).
  ○ Inferior turbinate hypertrophy requiring reduction in patients who have failed medical therapy.

TABLE 3-2	WHEN TO REFER TO AN ALLERGIST

Rhinitis with prolonged, severe disease and comorbid conditions such as:
- Asthma
- Recurrent sinusitis
- Nasal polyps

Complications occur
Patient has required systemic steroids for treatment
Symptoms interfere with quality of life or ability to function
Current medications are:
- Ineffective
- Associated with adverse reactions
- Multiple or costly over a prolonged period

Rhinitis medicamentosa has been diagnosed
Specific allergic triggers need identification
Increased level of education is desired
Allergen immunotherapy is considered
More education is needed
Patient requests consultation

○ Adenoid hypertrophy (adenoidectomy).
○ Nasal polyps which require removal (polypectomy).
○ Patients with complications from refractory rhinosinusitis (functional endoscopic sinus surgery).

MONITORING/FOLLOW-UP

- Clinical improvement is a better measure for appropriate environmental control than the amount of allergen concentration.[1]
- Patients should be assessed 2–4 weeks after initiation of therapy.[5]
  ○ Single-agent therapy with intranasal steroids or combination therapy with intranasal steroids and oral antihistamines is usually a good starting point.
  ○ Oral antihistamines should be tried before leukotriene inhibitors.[3]
  ○ Intranasal antihistamines and leukotrienes are more appropriate for those with seasonal AR.[3]
  ○ If one medication regimen does not seem to be effective, addition of an agent or change to a different class may be warranted.

SINUSITIS

GENERAL PRINCIPLES

- Normal sinus function requires:
  ○ All sinus ostia must be patent.
  ○ Normal mucociliary function.
  ○ Normal local and systemic immune function.[2]
- Rhinitis and sinusitis often coexist and rhinitis often precedes sinusitis.[2,6]

Definition

Sinusitis is simply defined as **inflammation** of one or more of the paranasal sinuses.

Classification

- Sinusitis is classified as acute, chronic, or recurrent.
- No consensus standards exist for defining chronic rhinosinusitis (CRS) versus acute rhinosinusitis (ARS).
- **ARS** is generally defined as symptoms for ≤1 month.
  - ○ Nasal drainage must be purulent.[2]
  - ○ Of note, acute sinusitis may last up to 12 weeks per episode.[6]
- **CRS** consists of inflammation of the nasal passages lasting 12 weeks at a minimum despite medical management.[2]
- **Recurrent sinusitis** is characterized by >4 episodes of acute sinusitis per year.[6] Patients with recurrent sinusitis may need evaluation for immunodeficiency.

Epidemiology

- Ninety to ninety-eight percent of episodes of sinusitis are preceded by an acute viral upper respiratory infection.[1]
- About 31 million people in the US have rhinosinusitis annually.[2]
- Prevalence is estimated at 10–30% in Europe and 15% in America.[6]
- **Viral upper respiratory infections become bacterial rhinosinusitis only in 0.5–2% of the population.**[2]
- Chronic sinusitis is associated with AR in 60% of adults.[2]
- Increasing resistance to first-line therapies is well known and includes β-lactamase production (gram-negative organisms) and alterations in penicillin-binding proteins (gram-positive organisms).
- More than one-third of *Haemophilus influenza* strains and virtually all *Moraxella catarrhalis* strains are penicillin resistant.

Etiology

- ARS is usually infectious, viral, bacterial, or fungal.[2]
  - ○ **Viruses** are the most common cause of acute sinusitis.
  - ○ The most common **bacterial** etiologies in acute sinusitis are the following:
    - *Streptococcus pneumoniae*
    - *H. influenza*
    - *M. catarrhalis*
- *Staphylococcus aureus,* coagulase-negative *Staphylococcus,* and anaerobic bacteria are more common in CRS, but **CRS is more often inflammatory.**[2]
- *S. aureus* is increasing in prevalence in sinusitis patients with nasal polyps.[2]
- *Pseudomonas aeruginosa* frequently occurs in patients with cystic fibrosis.
- Sinusitis is less commonly a manifestation of systemic illness.

Pathophysiology

- Acute sinusitis often develops when the sinus ostia are obstructed leading to infection.
- Conditions that **disrupt mucociliary clearance** of secretions and **promote ostial obstruction** predispose patients to sinusitis including:
  - ○ Rhinitis:
    - Ostial narrowing secondary to mucosal inflammation due to a viral infection.
    - Chronic mucosal changes from allergic disease.
  - ○ Nasal polyps.
  - ○ Anatomic abnormalities.

○ Foreign bodies.
○ Problems with mucociliary transport:
  ■ Cystic fibrosis.
  ■ Primary ciliary dyskinesia.
  ■ Viral infections and other causes of inflammation may also result in ciliary dysfunction.

DIAGNOSIS

Clinical Presentation

- The diagnosis of rhinosinusitis is usually entirely clinical and the differentiation between viral and bacterial infections can be difficult.
- Multiple studies regarding the utility of symptoms and signs for diagnosing acute sinusitis have sometimes reached differing conclusions. A few have used the true gold standard (i.e., sinus puncture and culture), but more have used a surrogate standard (e.g., sinus plain films and CT). Radiography cannot differentiate viral from bacterial sinusitis.
- ARS symptoms within the first 7–10 days of illness typically indicate a viral rhinosinusitis.[2]
- Regarding ARS, The American Academy of Allergy, Asthma, and Immunology (AAAAI) states the following (strength of recommendation level C):[7]
  ○ Acute bacterial rhinosinusitis may be suspected when an upper respiratory tract infection last longer than 10–14 days.
  ○ Bacterial infection is more likely with a history of persistent purulent rhinorrhea, postnasal drainage, and facial pain.
  ○ The prominent symptoms of acute bacterial rhinosinusitis are nasal congestion, purulent rhinorrhea, facial-dental pain, postnasal drainage, headache, and cough.
  ○ Signs of ARS include sinus tenderness, purulent nasal discharge, erythematous mucosa, pharyngeal secretions, and periorbital edema.
- The American Academy of Otolaryngology-Head and Neck Surgery guideline indicates that ARS may be diagnosed by the presence of one or both of the following:[8]
  ○ Up to 4 weeks of purulent nasal discharge accompanied by nasal obstruction.
  ○ Facial pain-pressure-fullness.
  ○ Acute bacterial (rather than viral) rhinosinusitis is diagnosed when:
    ■ Symptoms or signs persist ≥10 days after the onset of upper respiratory symptoms or
    ■ Symptoms or signs worsen within 10 days after an initial improvement.
- The American College of Physicians' clinical practice guideline advises the clinical diagnosis of acute bacterial rhinosinusitis should be made in those who:[9]
  ○ Have symptoms lasting ≥7 days and
  ○ Have maxillary pain or tenderness in the face or teeth and
  ○ Purulent nasal secretions.
- Two or more of the following symptoms when present are helpful when making the diagnosis of CRS in the setting of documented mucosal inflammation:[2]
  ○ Mucopurulent nasal drainage (anterior and/or posterior).
  ○ Nasal obstruction or blockage.
  ○ Facial pain, pressure, and/or fullness.
  ○ Decreased sense of smell.

TABLE 3-3	DIFFERENTIAL DIAGNOSIS FOR SINUSITIS

Viral upper respiratory infection
Rhinitis
Nonallergic rhinitis with eosinophilia syndrome (NARES)
Aspirin sensitivity
Nasal polyposis
Allergic fungal sinusitis
Infectious fungal sinusitis
Anatomic variants
Tumors
Foreign bodies
CSF rhinorrhea
Immunodeficiency
Wegener's granulomatosis
Cystic fibrosis
Kartagener's syndrome
Orbital cellulitis
Cavernous vein thrombosis
Meningitis
Brain abscess

Differential Diagnosis

- The differential diagnosis for rhinosinusitis is presented in Table 3-3.
- **Allergic fungal sinusitis:**
  - Rare cause of chronic sinusitis.
  - The hallmark feature is the presence of sinus opacification due to accumulation of "allergic mucin" that is thick, inspissated secretions heavily laden with eosinophils, Charcot–Leyden crystals, and fungal hyphae.
  - Diagnosis usually requires surgery to establish.[2]
- **Infectious fungal sinusitis:**
  - More likely to be seen in immunocompromised patients.
  - *Aspergillus fumigatus* is the most common cause of fungal sinusitis.

Diagnostic Testing

Laboratories
If **immunodeficiency** is suspected, obtain a complete blood count (CBC) with differential and quantitative immunoglobulin levels. Otherwise blood tests are of little use.

Imaging
- Imaging to confirm the diagnosis of acute uncomplicated rhinosinusitis is usually not necessary.[2,7–9]
- Radiography cannot readily differentiate viral from bacterial acute sinusitis.
- The limited sinus CT has become the most widely used radiographic study for the diagnosis of sinusitis.
  - It is obtained in the coronal projection with cuts through the frontal sinus, anterior ethmoid/maxillary sinuses, and posterior ethmoid and sphenoid sinuses.
  - Allows for assessment of patency of the osteomeatal unit, the critical confluence of drainage from the maxillary and anterior ethmoid sinuses.

- Imaging studies with CT usually reveal mucosal thickening and ostial plugging if the sinusitis is chronic.
  - CT is the test of choice for chronic sinusitis.[2]
- MRI is useful for evaluating allergic or infectious fungal sinusitis to rule out soft tissue extension.
  - It is not good for evaluating mucosal thickening or bony deformities.
  - Should not be used as an initial imaging method.

Diagnostic Procedures
- **Skin prick testing** evaluate for underlying AR may be performed.[2]
- **Edoscopically directed middle meatus cultures** may be helpful in adults.[1]
- **Rhinoscopy** with the flexible fiber optic rhinoscope can help determine nasal and sinus anatomy.
- **Biopsy** is indicated if there is suspicion of a tumor or vasculitis. A biopsy may also be helpful to confirm the presence of invasive fungal infection.
- **Ciliary function testing** is indicated in the setting of recurrent otitis, sinusitis, and pneumonia with bronchiectasis (primary ciliary dyskinesia or Kartagener's syndrome).
  - It is possible to do ciliary visual assessments, but a practical approach in the office setting is the **saccharine test.**
  - Electron microscopy of nasal mucosal biopsy is the only way to document abnormal cilia structure.
- **Nasal cytology:**
  - Presence of eosinophils may indicate AR, NARES, aspirin sensitivity, or nasal polyps.
  - Neutrophils are more indicative of infection.

TREATMENT

- Most cases of ARS are caused by viruses and are expected to significantly improve without antibiotic treatment within 10–14 days. Treatment should, therefore, be symptomatic for those without clinical signs suggestive of a bacterial infection.[7]
- Trials of the efficacy of antibiotics in ARS have been of variable quality and differing outcome measures. Most of the randomized trials did not definitively enroll only subjects with bacterial infections. Nonetheless, taken together, there does appear to be a modest benefit from antibiotic treatment. Of significant note, many patients in the control/placebo groups did spontaneously improve (on average 80% improved vs. 90% with antibiotics).[10]
- Uncomplicated acute bacterial rhinosinusitis may be treated with or without antibiotics.[2,8–10]
  - Patients without severe or prolonged symptoms may be managed initially with symptomatic treatment alone and followed for resolution. Worsening of symptoms during this time should prompt a reconsideration of antibiotic therapy.
  - Those with initially severe symptoms or those with symptoms for >7 days after diagnosis are typically treated with antibiotics.
  - Individual clinical judgment should be exercised when making the decision to forgo or prescribe antibiotic therapy.
- Appropriate first-line antibiotics for uncomplicated acute bacterial rhinosinusitis include amoxicillin, sulfamethoxazole-trimethoprim, and azithromycin for 10–14

days.[2,7–11] Significant differences between groups of antibiotics, including newer more expensive ones, have not been demonstrated.[8,10–12]

- The optimal duration of antibiotic therapy is unclear.[7]
- Alternative antibiotic therapy should be considered in patients who worsen or do not improve during the initial 7 days of therapy.[2,7,8,11] Reasonable second-line choices include high-dose amoxicillin–clavulanate, and oral fluoroquinolones and second- or third-generation cephalosporins.
- While evidence is somewhat limited, the addition of intranasal steroids may have modest positive benefit in the treatment of ARS.[2,7,13]
- There are no controlled trials of systemic steroids, and these are not routinely recommended.
- Analgesics should be prescribed to those with significant pain.[8]
- Data to support the use of decongestants, antihistamines, mucolytics/expectorants, and sinus irrigation are lacking, but they are at least theoretically beneficial and often recommended.[2,7]
- The treatment of CRS (i.e., ≥12 weeks), which is an inflammatory condition often accompanied by infection, is a more complicated matter. It may be associated with nasal polyposis or allergic fungal rhinosinusitis, or neither. Multicomponent treatment is necessary.
  - Intranasal steroids are generally recommended for all patients.[2,14] Oral steroids are sometimes used for severe symptoms.
  - Data regarding the use of antimicrobials in CRS are sparse; however, the potential for an infectious contribution to chronic inflammation seems clear. When there is an evidence of purulence, most clinician will treat with an antibiotic. On the basis of microbiologic studies, amoxicillin–clavulanate, clindamycin, or an oral fluoroquinolone are reasonable choices.[2,7,15] Duration of treatment is unclear, but 3 weeks is often recommended.
  - Nasal irrigation is frequently recommended.[16]
  - Patients with AR should be maximally treated as needed.
  - Surgical polypectomy may be indicated for severe polyposis.
  - Functional endoscopic sinus surgery is frequently done for refractory CRS.

COMPLICATIONS

- Rare but dangerous complications may occur when sinus disease extends outside of the sinus cavity. These include orbital cellulitis, cavernous vein thrombosis, brain abscess, meningitis, osteomyelitis, oral-antral fistula, and mucocele.[2,6]
- It should be remembered that *Clostridium difficile* colitis and candidiasis can be a complication of prolonged antibiotic therapy.

REFERRAL

Indications for referral to an ENT surgeon are as follows:[1,2,6]

- Evidence of anatomic defects by CT or physical examination, including foreign bodies, and tumors.
- Nasal polyps that obstruct sinus drainage despite medical treatment.
- Persistent sinusitis despite aggressive medical management.
- Sinus condition requiring biopsy.
- Sinusitis complicated by extension into local structures.

MONITORING/FOLLOW-UP

- Symptoms are expected to resolve between episodes of ARS.
- If symptoms continue after one course of antibiotics, an alternative antibiotic may be considered.
- If symptoms have not resolved after multiple courses of antibiotics, CT scan should be performed, and further workup for predisposing conditions should be performed.

REFERENCES

1. Wallace DV, Dykewicz MS, Bernstein DI, et al. The diagnosis and management of rhinitis: an updated practice parameter. *J Allergy Clin Immunol.* 2008;122:S1–S84.
2. Dykewicz MS, Hamilos DL. Rhinitis and sinusitis. *J Allergy Clin Immunol.* 2010;125: S103–S115.
3. Brozek JL, Bousquet J, Baena-Cagnani CE, et al. Allergic rhinitis and its impact on asthma (ARIA) guidelines: 2010 revision. *J Allergy Clin Immunol.* 2010;126:466–476.
4. Harvey R, Hannan SA, Badia L, et al. Nasal saline irrigations for the symptoms of chronic rhinosinusitis. *Cochran Database Syst Rev.* 2007;(3):CD006394.
5. Price D, Bond C, Bouchard J, et al. International primary care respiratory group (IPCRG) guidelines: management of allergic rhinitis. *Prim Care Respir. J.* 2006;15:58–70.
6. Bachert C, Gevaert P, Cauwenberge P. Nasal polyps and rhinosinusitis. In: Adkinson NF, Holgate ST, Bochner BS, et al., eds. *Middleton's Allergy: Principles and Practice,* 7th ed. Philadelphia, PA: Mosby/Elsevier, 2009:995–1004.
7. Slavin RG, Spector SL, Bernstein IL, et al. The diagnosis and management of sinusitis: a practice parameter update. *J Allergy Clin Immunol.* 2005;116:S13–S47.
8. Rosenfeld RM. Clinical practice guideline on adult sinusitis. *Otolaryngol Head Neck Surg.* 2007;137:365–377.
9. Hickner JM, Bartlett JG, Besser RE, et al. Principles of appropriate antibiotic use for acute rhinosinusitis in adults: background. *Ann Intern Med.* 2001;134:498–505.
10. Ahovuo-Saloranta A, Borisenko OV, Kovanen N, et al. Antibiotics for acute maxillary sinusitis. *Cochrane Database Syst Rev.* 2008;(2):CD000243.
11. Piccirillo JF. Acute bacterial sinusitis. *N Engl J Med.* 2004;351:902–910.
12. Piccirillo JF, Mage DE, Frisse ME, et al. Impact of first-line vs second-line antibiotics for the treatment of acute uncomplicated sinusitis. *JAMA.* 2001;286:1849–1856.
13. Zalmanovici A, Yaphe J. Intranasal steroids for acute sinusitis. *Cochrane Database Syst Rev.* 2009;(4):CD005149.
14. Snidvongs K, Kalish L, Sacks R, et al. Topical steroid for chronic rhinosinusitis without polyps. *Cochrane Database Syst Rev.* 2011;(8):CD009274.
15. Piromchai P, Thanaviratananich S, Laopaiboon M. Systemic antibiotics for chronic rhinosinusitis without nasal polyps in adults. *Cochrane Database Syst Rev.* 2011;(5):CD008233.
16. Harvey R, Hannan SA, Badia L, et al. Nasal saline irrigations for the symptoms of chronic rhinosinusitis. *Cochrane Database Syst Rev.* 2007;(3):CD006394.

Asthma

4

Natalie Miller and Sarena Sawlani

GENERAL PRINCIPLES

Definition

- Asthma is a **chronic inflammatory disorder of the airways associated with airway hyperresponsiveness,** which leads to recurrent wheezing, coughing, and difficulty breathing.[1]
- **Variable, reversible airflow obstruction** is a hallmark of asthma. Reversibility can either be spontaneous or with treatment.
- **Asthma exacerbations** are periods of worsening symptom between periods of relative symptom stability.
- Most childhood asthma is the result of atopic sensitization and is considered part of the allergic diathesis.
- Adult-onset asthma can not only be part of the spectrum of atopy but can also result from other etiologies, such as occupational exposures.

Classification

Asthma classification is based on symptom severity at diagnosis (Table 4-1), control at follow-up visits and severity/frequency of exacerbations (Table 4-2) (e.g., "moderate persistent asthma currently well controlled").[2]

Epidemiology

- As of 2005, an estimated 32.6 million Americans (11.2% total population) have a diagnosis of asthma sometime during their lifetime.[1]
- Asthma prevalence has increased from 7.3 to 8.2% from 2001 to 2009.[3]
  - On the basis of 2004 estimate, approximately 300 million people of all ages suffered from asthma. By 2025, it is also expected that over 400 million people will suffer from the disease per the Global Initiative for Asthma (GINA).[4]
  - A correlation has been noted between the increase of asthma prevalence with **atopic sensitization,** which can be seen by the increase of allergic rhinitis and eczema.[4,5]
  - Asthma is a worldwide disorder but more common in developed countries (e.g., Australia, New Zealand, US, Ireland, UK).
  - The **hygiene hypothesis** (see Chapter 2) suggests that the rising prevalence of asthma in developed countries is due to the overall decrease in viral and bacterial infections, which increase activation of Th2 lymphocytes, which is associated with asthma and atopy. Also, the increased use of antibiotic in children may alter the normal gut flora in infants and increase the Th2 immune response.
  - Multiple studies have hypothesized that specific **air pollutants** have been linked to asthma.[6,7]

TABLE 4-1 CLASSIFICATION OF ASTHMA SEVERITY[a]

Components of severity		Intermittent	Mild (Persistent)	Moderate (Persistent)	Severe (Persistent)
Impairment	Symptoms	≤2 days/week	>2 days/week but not daily	Daily	Throughout the day
	Nighttime awakenings	≤2×/month	3–4×/month	>1×/week but not nightly	Often 7×/week
	SABA use for symptom control (not prevention of EIB)	≤2 days/week	>2 days/week but not daily and not more than 1× on any day	Daily	Several times per day
	Interference with normal activity	None	Minor limitation	Some limitation	Extremely limited
	Lung function[b]	Normal FEV$_1$ between exacerbations FEV$_1$ >80% predicted FEV$_1$/FVC normal	FEV$_1$ >80% predicted FEV$_1$/FVC normal	FEV$_1$ >60% but <80% predicted FEV$_1$/FVC reduced 5%	FEV$_1$ <60% predicted FEV$_1$/FVC reduced >5%
Risk	Exacerbations requiring oral systemic corticosteroids	0–1/year	≥2/year	≥2/year	≥2/year
Recommended starting step (see Fig. 4-1)		Step 1	Step 2	Step 3	Step 4 or 5 Consider short course of OSC

Adapted from: Summary Report 2007. National Institutes of Health. National Heart, Lung, and Blood Institute. National Asthma Education and Prevention Program Expert Panel Report 3 (EPR-3): Guidelines for the Diagnosis and Management of Asthma. NIH Publication 08-5846, Bethesda, MD, August 2007.

SABA, short-acting β$_2$-agonist; EIB, exercise-induced bronchospasm; FVC, forced vital capacity; FEV$_1$, forced expiratory volume at 1 second; OSC, oral systemic corticosteroids.

[a]For patients ≥12 years old.

[b]Normal FEV$_1$/FVC: 8–19 years old, 85%; 20–39 years old, 80%; 40–59 years old, 75%; 60–80 years old, 70%.

TABLE 4-2 CLASSIFICATION OF ASTHMA CONTROL[a]

		Classification of asthma control		
Components of control		**Well controlled**	**Not well controlled**	**Very poorly controlled**
Impairment	Symptoms	≤2 days/week	>2 days/week	Throughout the day
	Nighttime awakenings	≤2×/month	1–3×/week	≥4×/week
	Interference with normal activity	None	Some limitation	Extremely limited
	SABA use for symptom control (not prevention of EIB)	≤2 days/week	>2 days/week	Several times per day
	FEV₁ or peak flow	>80% predicted/ personal best	60–80% predicted/ personal best	<60% predicted/ personal best
	Validated questionnaires:			
	ATAQ	0	1–2	3–4
	ACQ	≤0.75	≥1.5	N/A
	ACT	≥20	16–19	≤15
Risk	Exacerbations requiring oral systemic corticosteroids	0–1/year	≥2/year	≥2/year
	Progressive loss of lung function	Evaluation requires long-term follow-up care		
	Treatment-related adverse effects	Medication side effects can vary in intensity from none to very troublesome and worrisome. The level of intensity does not correlate to specific levels of control but should be considered in the overall assessment of risk.		

Adapted from: Summary Report 2007. National Institutes of Health. National Heart, Lung, and Blood Institute. National Asthma Education and Prevention Program Expert Panel Report 3 (EPR-3): Guidelines for the Diagnosis and Management of Asthma. NIH Publication 08-5846, Bethesda, MD, August 2007.

SABA, short-acting β₂-agonist; EIB, exercise-induced bronchospasm; FEV₁, forced expiratory volume at 1 second; ATAQ, asthma therapy assessment questionnaire; ACQ, asthma control questionnaire; ACT, asthma control test.

[a]For patients ≥12 years old.

- Exposure to **nitrogen dioxide** along with living in close proximity (<50 m distance) to a major road has been associated with higher rates of asthma risk and incidents.[8]
- Chronic exposure to nitrogen dioxide from indoor gas stoves may be associated with increase in asthma symptoms found in lower socioeconomic groups.[9]
- **Diesel fuel exhaust** particles have also been hypothesized to be taken up by epithelial cells in the airway leading to allergic immune responses.[10]
- **Socioeconomic considerations:**
  - A higher rate of asthma prevalence has been seen in blacks than in whites.[11]
  - In people living in poverty and the inner city, increased asthma prevalence and mortality may be associated with the lack of adherence to asthma treatment complicated by a decreased or lack of access to medical care or insurance.[12]
  - Other risk factors include low birth weight secondary to maternal tobacco use and tobacco exposure in the home.
  - In 2004, there were nearly half a million hospitalizations; 190,000 of these were below age 15. Blacks were 3.4 times more likely than whites to be hospitalized.
- Mortality from asthma is relatively rare and has declined since 1999 to four deaths per million.
  - The US initially had an increase in the annual death rate between the years 1982 and 1995. However, since then, the death rate has decreased.[11]
  - Deaths are higher in blacks, in all age groups, compared to whites.
- **Risk factors for fatal asthma** in patients include major and minor risk factors.
  - Major risk factors include:
    - A recent history of poorly controlled asthma (e.g., increase in daily and/or nocturnal awakening due to shortness of breath or wheezing, increased use of β_2-agonist, and variation of peak flow results).
    - A history of a near fatal episode of asthma (intensive care unit admission and/or requirement of intubation previously).
  - Minor risk factors include aeroallergen exposure, aspirin/nonsteroidal anti-inflammatory drug (NSAID) exposure, cigarette smoke, illicit drug use, genetic factors, multiple emergency department visits or admissions for asthma, multiple oral glucocorticosteroid requirements, and poor medical adherence.

Pathophysiology

- The pathogenesis of asthma is complex and results from a combination of factors including **genetic, environmental, immunologic, and developmental factors.** Furthermore, asthma is likely a heterogeneous disease with **multiple pathways leading to airway hyperresponsiveness.** Nevertheless, airway narrowing causing obstruction of airflow results in **bronchoconstriction, which is the dominant physiologic event leading to clinical symptoms.**[13]
- **Airway inflammation** is an important factor predisposing to bronchoconstriction.
  - Immunoglobulin E (IgE)-mediated inflammation is caused by antigen-mediated crosslinking of IgE on the surface of mast cells resulting in the release of inflammatory mediators (see Chapter 2).
  - Non–IgE-mediated inflammation in asthma is less well understood but ultimately results in airway edema and inflammation. There are multiple subtypes defined including aspirin-sensitive asthma and neutrophilic asthma.
- Airway diameter is decreased by edema, inflammation, increase in mucous secretion (which, in turn, can lead to mucous plugging), and structural changes.

- Airway hyperresponsiveness can result from exaggerated bronchoconstriction due to inflammation, neuroregulatory dysfunction, and structural changes. Bronchoconstriction can be triggered in response to various stimuli including tobacco smoke, weather changes, or emotions.
- Permanent structural changes from chronic inflammation result in progressive loss of lung function that is not completely reversible by therapy. Thickening of the sub-basement membrane, subepithelial fibrosis, airway smooth muscle hypertrophy, mucous gland hypertrophy, and hypersecretion all contribute to these changes.

Risk Factors

- **Atopy:** Epidemiologic studies consistently show an association between atopic sensitization and asthma, but the causal relationship is complex.[1]
- **Genetics:** A combination of genetic susceptibility and an appropriate environmental stimulus causes asthma. Genome-wide association studies have identified over 100 genes associated with asthma. The studies suggest that a complex interaction of genes combined with environmental exposure(s) results in asthma.
  - Parental diagnosis of asthma increases the risk of asthma in an offspring.
  - Twin studies show higher concordance rates in monozygotic twins.
- **Gender:** In early childhood, male children are at a greater risk for developing asthma, while in adolescents and adulthood females are at greater risk.
- **Prematurity** has been associated with the development of symptoms consistent with asthma, both with and without a history of neonatal respiratory distress, but the mechanism and its involvement with other asthma risk factors are not known.
- **Passive tobacco smoke exposure:** *In utero* exposure to tobacco smoke affects airway responsiveness after birth. Children exposed to secondhand smoke have an increased frequency of wheezing and increased risk of more severe lower respiratory tract infection during the first year of life.
- **Respiratory infections,** especially respiratory syncytial virus and parainfluenza, have been associated with childhood wheezing. While follow-up studies are suggestive of a relationship with developing asthma, definitive evidence is still lacking. Respiratory infections are associated with asthma exacerbations.
- **The Asthma predictive index** was established from the evaluation of risk factor for persistent asthma and predicts development of persistent asthma after 6 years of age.[2]
  - Recurrent wheezing in children 3 years of age or younger, and
  - One major criterion (parental asthma or physician diagnosed eczema in patient) or
  - Two minor criteria (eosinophilia >4%, wheezing without colds, allergic rhinitis)

Prevention

- Identify **precipitating factors** such as exposure to allergens, irritants, and viruses, and **limiting exposure** to these triggering factors is key to preventing asthma exacerbations.[2]
- **Treatment of other comorbidities** that can worsen asthma should be optimized to reduce morbidity from asthma (e.g., conditions such as allergic rhinitis, sleep apnea, sinusitis, and gastroesophageal reflux disease).
- **Smoking cessation** must be a priority for any individual with asthma.

Associated Conditions

- Atopic diseases, including food allergy, eczema, and allergic rhinitis, are frequently comorbid with asthma.

- The **atopic march** denotes the successive development of food allergy, eczema, allergic rhinitis, and asthma in childhood.
- **Samter's triad** is the co-occurrence of asthma, nasal polyps, and aspirin sensitivity.

DIAGNOSIS

Clinical Presentation

History

- The hallmark of asthma is recurrent episodes of **reversible bronchoconstriction.**
- Asthma exacerbations can manifest with:
  - **Shortness of breath** that is typically worsened with exertion.
  - **Chest tightness** or pain.
  - **Wheezing** which may be audible to the patient or caregiver, but often time is not.
  - **Cough** that is often productive of inspissated secretions without being related to an infection cause.
    - Some patients rarely wheeze but cough instead, especially children. This is an important feature that should not be missed, because patients with **cough-variant asthma** generally respond well to therapy but often go undiagnosed.
    - Marked dyspnea and agitation in a patient who can speak in full sentences should cause one to consider **vocal cord dysfunction** (VCD).
    - Curschmann's spirals are helical mucous plugs often observed in asthmatic's sputum.
- **Nocturnal awakenings** with coughing or wheezing may be the presenting symptom, especially in children. Nocturnal symptoms in a patient who has previously had only daytime symptoms represent disease progression.
- **Exercise-induced bronchospasm** may also be the presenting symptom. Consider asthma if a child cannot keep up with peers during athletic activity secondary to coughing or wheezing.
- Family history is frequently notable for the presence of atopic diseases.
- Asthma triggers such as exercise, viral infections, environmental triggers, smoke, should be identified during the history.
- Environmental history should be carefully reviewed for potential allergen exposures and should include:
  - Details about the home/work/school environment
  - Whether the patient has a seasonal or perennial profile of symptoms
  - Animal exposure
  - Smoking history

Physical Examination

- Between acute exacerbations, asthmatic patients may have a completely normal physical examination.
- Vital signs can be normal, even during an acute exacerbation. Elevated heart rate and respiratory rate are the most frequent abnormalities. Oxygen desaturation tends to be a late sign in adults and indicates impending respiratory failure.
- General appearance can be an important indicator of severity. **Inability to speak in complete sentences, agitation, or lethargy are alarming signs** and should prompt immediate intervention.
- Examination of the head, eyes, ears, nose, and throat may show signs of allergic disease or accessory muscle usage (especially in children). **Stridor or wheezing best heard in the neck suggests an alternative diagnosis** such as VCD or upper airway obstruction.

TABLE 4-3	DIFFERENTIAL DIAGNOSES OF ADULT ASTHMA
COPD	Mechanical upper airway obstruction:
Congestive heart failure	Tumor
Pulmonary embolism	Epiglottitis
Tracheomalacia	VCD
Pulmonary eosinophilia	Foreign body
ABPA	Obstructive sleep apnea
Allergic rhinitis	

COPD, chronic obstructive pulmonary disease; VCD, vocal cord dysfunction; ABPA, Allergic bronchopulmonary aspergillosis.

- The lung examination frequently demonstrates high-pitched end expiratory wheezing. **In severe asthma exacerbations, wheezing may not be heard** at all and may indicate impending respiratory failure.
  - Rhonchi or focal findings suggest a pulmonary infection that may have triggered the exacerbation or, in the absence of fever, may represent the tenacious secretions commonly seen in asthmatics.
  - Respiratory muscle alternans is the paradoxical movement of the diaphragm with alternating abdominal and ribcage breathing. It represents a patient in extremis and is more commonly seen in children.
- Other examination findings may include:
  - Intercostal retractions may be present during an exacerbation, particularly in children.
  - Signs of Cushing's syndrome secondary to exogenous steroid use.
  - Symptoms of other comorbid atopic conditions such as eczema.

Differential Diagnosis
- The differential diagnosis of asthma in adults is presented in Table 4-3.
- **VCD** is voluntary or involuntary adduction of the true or false vocal cords resulting in dyspnea that can mimic asthma.
  - Up to 40% of asthmatics may exhibit VCD.
  - In addition to dyspnea, patients often present with a choking sensation, dysphonia, and cough.
  - Wheezing heard best at the larynx is suggestive of VCD.
  - Pulmonary function test (PFT) flow volume loops may show flattening of the inspiratory curve.
  - Diagnosis of VCD is made by direct visualization of the vocal cords showing paradoxical movement during respiration.
  - Treatment consists of speech therapy. Early diagnosis is important to avoid prolonged, unnecessary treatment, and some patients may also benefit from psychiatric counseling.

Diagnostic Testing
Laboratories
- Routine laboratory tests are usually normal in asthma but may demonstrate neutrophilia if the patient is on steroids.

- **Arterial blood gas measurement** may be indicated if a patient is in danger of respiratory failure.
  - Most patients will have a respiratory alkalosis from hyperventilation as the patient works to increase minute ventilation.
  - A patient whose CO_2 is normal or above normal during a severe exacerbation is in danger of respiratory failure. This "normal" value represents a patient who can no longer maintain a high minute ventilation and has begun to tire out.

Imaging
- An initial chest radiograph (CXR) of a pediatric patient who is wheezing for the first time is necessary to rule out aspiration of a foreign body.
- A CXR should also be obtained for any patient requiring admission.
- CXR is rarely necessary in the outpatient setting for an established asthmatic.
- CXR may demonstrate:
  - Hyperinflation (flattening of the diaphragms).
  - Mucous plugging (linear atelectasis).
  - These findings may be indistinguishable from chronic obstructive pulmonary disease (COPD).
- CXR is particularly useful in patients who present with new-onset wheezing, have other comorbidities (e.g., congestive heart failure, COPD, or pneumonia), or have focal findings on examination.
- One should also obtain a CXR when suspicion of a pneumothorax or pneumomediastinum is present.

Diagnostic Procedures
- **PFT** is an important component of asthma management (see Chapter 7).
  - While there is no single, definitive diagnostic test for asthma, demonstration of reversible airway obstruction strongly supports the diagnosis.
  - Methacholine challenge can be used to demonstrate airway hyperresponsiveness when the question of asthma is in question.
- **Aeroallergen skin testing** (see Chapter 8) will demonstrate positivity to one or more allergens in atopic asthma and is often useful in guiding therapy and counseling on allergen avoidance.

TREATMENT

- Long-term goals for the management of asthma include reduction of risk and impairment.[2]
- Reduce risk of morbidity and mortality by:
  - Preventing exacerbations and minimizing emergency department visits/hospitalizations.
  - Preventing permanent loss of lung function.
  - Minimizing side effects of pharmacotherapy.
- Reduce functional impairment by:
  - Preventing day-to-day symptoms including coughing or shortness of breath.
  - Minimizing use (≤ 2 days/week) of short-acting β_2-agonists (SABAs) for relief of symptoms (excluding pre-treatment for exercise-induced asthma).
  - Maintaining normal activity levels to minimize interruption of exercise and attendance at work/school.

Medications

Short-acting Medications

- **SABAs,** such as albuterol or levalbuterol, are inhaled medications that work through airway β_2 receptors to relax the airway smooth muscle.
  - Used in all types of asthma for relief of acute symptoms.
  - Also indicated for use as pre-treatment in exercise-induced asthma.
- **Anticholinergics** inhibit muscarinic cholinergic receptors and reduce intrinsic airway vagal tone leading to bronchodilation.
  - Generally considered to be less effective in treating asthma symptoms than SABAs.
  - Most commonly used in combination with a SABA for moderate to severe asthma exacerbations and for those individuals who do not tolerate SABA (e.g., tachyarrhythmias).
- **Systemic corticosteroids** are administered either parenterally or orally and are perhaps the most potent anti-inflammatory medications used to treat asthma.
  - Primary indication in asthma is to treat moderate to severe exacerbations.
  - Systemic steroids should be reserved for asthma exacerbations with every effort made to transition to long-term controller medications.
  - A small subset of severe asthmatics with steroid-dependent asthma are unable to tolerate withdrawal of steroids because of severe respiratory symptoms.
  - The side effects of corticosteroids are multifold and include neuropsychiatric disturbances, weight gain, glucose intolerance, increased susceptibility to infections, avascular necrosis, growth stunting, and adrenal insufficiency when used chronically.

Long-term Control Medications

- **Inhaled corticosteroids (ICSs) are mainstays of persistent asthma therapy.**
  - They are primarily anti-inflammatory, blocking late-phase reaction to allergen, reducing airway hyperresponsiveness and inhibiting inflammatory cell migration and activation.
  - ICSs have an onset of action of several days, and their **maximal activity is seen 2–3 weeks after initiation of therapy.** Therefore, ICSs should not be used as rescue medications.
  - Local side effects include dysphonia, throat irritation, and oral candidiasis. Mouth rinsing after inhaler use may help prevent thrush.
  - Systemic side effects from ICSs are minimal in adults because of first-pass metabolism in the liver.
    - Adrenal suppression is theoretically possible, but the risk of symptomatic adrenal suppression is very small.
    - There is no clear link of ICSs to increased risk of osteoporosis. Nevertheless, clinicians should consider screening individuals at risk for osteoporosis who also need ICSs.
    - In children, ICSs are linked to a slightly delayed growth velocity. This effect is considered transient, as it does not affect the final adult height.
- **Long-acting β_2-agonists (LABAs)** are long-acting inhaled medications that are capable of providing bronchodilation for at least 12 hours (e.g., salmeterol and formoterol).
  - Studies have suggested increased mortality associated with LABA, though this seems to be associated with LABA monotherapy.
  - **LABAs should not be used as monotherapy, only as adjunctive therapy with ICS for control of moderate persistent or severe persistent asthma.**[14]
- **Leukotriene modifiers** are medications that alter the signaling or synthesis of leukotrienes, which are lipid inflammatory mediators.

○ Leukotriene receptor antagonists (LTRAs) (montelukast and zafirlukast) and a 5-lipoxygenase inhibitor (zileuton) are commercially available.
○ They may be particularly effective in **aspirin-sensitive asthma** as well as **exercise-induced asthma**.
- **Mast cell stabilizers** act by preventing degranulation of mast cells.
  ○ Generally, these are older, less effective medications, and as such, they are considered alternative treatments for mild persistent asthma.
  ○ Cromolyn sodium and nedocromil are examples of mast cell stabilizers.
- **Theophylline** is a methylxanthine drug that functions both as a phosphodiesterase inhibitor and an adenosine receptor antagonist to stimulate bronchodilation and reduce airway inflammation.
  ○ Serum levels of theophylline must be measured periodically as it has a relatively narrow therapeutic range. Normal levels are 5–15 μg/mL.
  ○ Serious side effects include cardiac arrhythmia and seizure.
- **Anti-IgE therapy** (i.e., omalizumab) is subcutaneously administered, humanized, monoclonal antibody against human IgE. Expense limits its usage to patients with moderate to severe asthma with demonstrated sensitivity to perennial allergens.

Asthma Management
- **Acute exacerbation management** (Table 4-4):[2]
- The focus of treatment is to immediately alleviate symptoms.
  ○ Frequent need for **oral corticosteroid**s should prompt re-evaluation of therapeutic management.
  ○ **Antibiotics** are not routinely indicated for exacerbations unless there are signs or symptoms of coincident infection.
  ○ Intravenous **magnesium sulfate** (2 g infused over 20 minutes) may provide some benefit for patients with severe exacerbations.[15,16]
- **Long-term management:**
  ○ A stepwise approach to increasing therapy is recommended (Fig. 4-1).
  ○ Asthma control should be reassessed periodically while on therapy and treatment tailored to the level of control (Table 4-2).[2]
  ○ Step-down therapy should be considered when asthma is well controlled to determine the minimum necessary medications.
  ○ **Patient education** is key to long-term asthma control.
    ■ Home **peak-flow monitoring** may be helpful in monitoring asthma control, especially in patients who have difficulty assessing their own symptoms.
    ■ **Asthma action plans** indicate a stepwise treatment plan tailored to each individual patient. Typically, they indicate warning signs of worsening symptoms such as a decrease in peak flow, along with a therapeutic intervention.
    ■ **Identify and recognize triggers** so that patients are able to implement environmental controls to reduce exacerbations.
  ○ **Yearly influenza vaccination** is recommended because asthmatic patients are more susceptible to complications.

COMPLICATIONS

Status Asthmaticus
- Defined as a severe exacerbation that fails to respond rapidly to sympathomimetic agents.

TABLE 4-4	ACUTE ASTHMA EXACERBATION MANAGEMENT		
	Symptoms and signs	Initial PEF (or FEV$_1$)	Clinical course
Mild	Dyspnea only with activity (assess tachypnea in young children)	PEF ≥70% predicted or personal best	• Usually cared for at home • Prompt relief with inhaled SABA • Possible short course of oral systemic corticosteroids
Moderate	Dyspnea interferes with or limits usual activity	PEF 40–69% predicted or personal best	• Usually requires office or ED visit • Relief from frequent inhaled SABA • OSC; some symptoms last for 1–2 days after treatment is begun
Severe	Dyspnea at rest; interferes with conversation	PEF <40% predicted or personal best	• Usually requires ED visit and likely hospitalization • Partial relief from frequent inhaled SABA • OSC; some symptoms last for >3 days after treatment is begun • Adjunctive therapies are helpful
Life-threatening	Too dyspneic to speak; perspiring	PEF <25% of predicted or personal best	• Requires ED/hospitalization; possible ICU • Minimal or no relief from frequent inhaled SABA • Intravenous corticosteroids • Adjunctive therapies are helpful

Adapted from: Summary Report 2007. National Institutes of Health. National Heart, Lung, and Blood Institute. National Asthma Education and Prevention Program Expert Panel Report 3 (EPR-3): Guidelines for the Diagnosis and Management of Asthma. NIH Publication 08-5846, Bethesda, MD, August 2007.

PEF, peak expiratory flow; FEV$_1$, forced expiratory volume at 1 second; SABA, short-acting β_2-agonist; ED, emergency department; OSC, oral systemic corticosteroid; ICU, intensive care unit.

• Patients at risk for status are those who are on oral steroids, who smoke, who have previously been intubated, who have been admitted to an intensive care unit within the last year, and who frequently or recently visited the emergency department.

Allergic Bronchopulmonary Aspergillosis

• Allergic bronchopulmonary aspergillosis (ABPA) is a rare complication of asthma and, more frequently, cystic fibrosis.

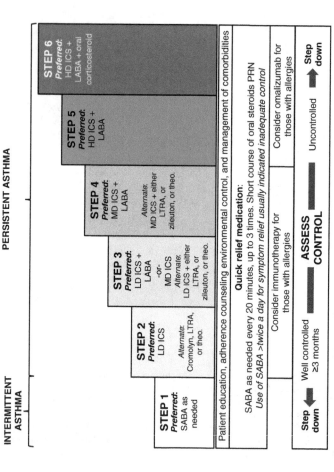

FIGURE 4-1 Stepwise asthma management. Adapted from: Summary Report 2007. National Institutes of Health. National Heart, Lung, and Blood Institute. National Asthma Education and Prevention Program Expert Panel Report 3 (EPR-3): Guidelines for the Diagnosis and Management of Asthma. NIH Publication 08-5846, Bethesda, MD, August 2007. HD, high dose; ICS, inhaled corticosteroid; LABA, long-acting β_2-agonist; LD, low dose; LTRA, leukotriene receptor antagonist; MD, medium dose; SABA, short-acting β-agonist; theo, theophylline.

- *Aspergillus fumigatus* is a common environmental mold that, in the immunocompromised host, can cause invasive infections. It is also a common allergen to which many atopic patients are sensitized that contributes to both asthma and allergic rhinitis.
- **ABPA represents colonization (rather than infection) with *Aspergillus* and subsequent development of *Aspergillus* hypersensitivity.** This results in bronchial inflammation, bronchiectasis, and respiratory complications.
- A small subset of patients who have asthma progresses to intractable ABPA and, often, oral corticosteroid–dependent disease.

SPECIAL CONSIDERATIONS

Asthma During Pregnancy

- Asthma control during pregnancy is variable with roughly one-third of women improving, one-third remaining stable, and one-third deteriorating.
- Very few medications have been investigated for their safety during pregnancy.
  - Budesonide is the only category B ICS (no evidence of risk to fetus).
  - SABAs appear to be relatively safe, though there may be a small teratogenic risk to the fetus.
  - There is very little experience with LABAs in pregnancy, though animal studies are reassuring.
  - High-dose systemic corticosteroids have been associated with congenital malformations and low birth weight.
- Poorly controlled asthma increases the risk to the fetus due to maternal hypoxia.
- Careful reassessment of asthma control medications before pregnancy and discussion with the patient is necessary to minimize risk to the fetus.

REFERENCES

1. Tang EA, Matsui E, Wiesch DG, et al. Epidemiology of asthma and allergic diseases. In: Adkinson NF, Bochner BS, Busse WW, et al., eds. *Middleton's Allergy: Principles and Practice*, 7th ed. Philadelphia, PA: Elsevier, 2009:715–756.
2. Summary Report 2007. National Institutes of Health. *National Heart, Lung, and Blood Institute. National Asthma Education and Prevention Program Expert Panel Report 3 (EPR-3): Guidelines for the Diagnosis and Management of Asthma. NIH Publication 08-5846*, Bethesda, MD, August 2007.
3. Centers for Disease Control Prevention (CDC). Vital signs: asthma prevalence, disease characteristics, and self-management education: United States, 2001–2009. *MMWR Morb Mort Wkly Rep.* 2011;60:547–552.
4. Masoli M, Fabian D, Holt S, et al. The global burden of asthma: executive summary of the GINA Dissemination Committee report. *Allergy.* 2004;59:469–478.
5. von Mutius E, Martinez FD, Fritzsch C, et al. Prevalence of asthma and atopy in two areas of West and East Germany. *Am J Respir Crit Care Med.* 1994;149:358–364.
6. Jin C, Shelburne CP, Li G, et al. Particulate allergens potentiate allergic asthma in mice through sustained IgE-mediated mast cell activation. *J Clin Invest.* 2011;121:3189–3205.
7. Magnussen H, Jörres R, Nowak D. Effect of air pollution on the prevalence of asthma and allergy: lessons from the German reunification. *Thorax.* 1993;48:879–885.
8. Modig L, Torén K, Janson C, et al. Vehicle exhaust outside the home and onset of asthma among adults. *Eur Respir J.* 2009;33:1261–1267.
9. Belanger K, Gent JF, Triche EW, et al. Association of indoor nitrogen dioxide exposure with respiratory symptoms in children with asthma. *Am J Respir Crit Care Med.* 2006;173:297–303.

10. Bleck B, Tse DB, Jaspers I, et al. Diesel exhaust particle-exposed human bronchial epithelial cell induce dendritic cell maturation. *J Immunol.* 2006;176:7431–7437.
11. Moorman JE, Rudd RA, Johnson CA, et al. National surveillance for asthma – United States, 1980–2004. *MMWR Surveill Summ.* 2007;56:1–54.
12. Weiss KB, Gergen PJ, Crain EF. Inner-city asthma. The epidemiology of an emerging US public health concern. *Chest.* 1992;101:362S–367S.
13. Holgate ST, Lemanske RF, O'Byrne PM, et al. *Asthma pathogenesis.* In: Adkinson NF, Bochner BS, Busse WW, et al., eds. *Middleton's Allergy: Principles and Practice,* 7th ed. Philadelphia, PA: Elsevier, 2007:893–915.
14. Tovey D. Asthma challenges: the place of inhaled long-acting beta-agonists. *Cochrane Database Syst Rev.* 2010;8:ED000002.
15. Silverman RA, Osborn H, Runge J, et al. IV magnesium sulfate in the treatment of acute severe asthma: a multicenter randomized controlled trial. *Chest.* 2002;122:489–497.
16. Rowe BH, Bretzlaff JA, Bourdon C, et al. Magnesium sulfate for treating exacerbations of acute asthma in the emergency department. *Cochrane Database Syst Rev.* 2000;(2):CD001490.

Occupational Asthma

5

Seema Mahale

GENERAL PRINCIPLES

Definition

- Occupational asthma (OA) is defined as variable airflow limitation and/or bronchial hyperresponsiveness caused by exposures in the work place setting.
- OA also includes preexistent asthma that is worsened when exposed to the work place.
- There are two types of OA:
  - **Sensitizer-induced OA**, previously known as latent OA.
  - **Irritant-induced OA**, previously known as nonlatent OA.

Classification

Sensitizer-induced Occupational Asthma

- Symptoms of asthma occur after a **latency period** of months to years after initial exposure to sensitizing substance in the work place.
- After the patient has been sensitized, airway reaction begins to develop at levels of sensitizer that were previously tolerable. **Typically, this is an immunologically mediated reaction.**
- Different types of sensitizers are categorized by size:
  - **High molecular weight (HMW)**: Agents >10 kD, **commonly inhaled proteins.**
  - **Low molecular weight (LMW)**: Agents <10 kD, **haptenated chemical.**

Irritant-induced Occupational Asthma

- Exposure to high levels of irritant agent can lead to **reactive airways dysfunction syndrome (RADS).**
- There is **no latent period**, and asthma symptoms occur within 24 hours of exposure to the irritant substance.
- Typical setting is an occupational accident that leads to exposure of unusually high levels of irritant.
- **Diagnosis cannot be made in patients with preexisting asthma.**

Epidemiology

- It is estimated that 15–25% of *de novo* adult asthma is due to work-related asthma.[1,2]
- Prevalence of OA is difficult to assess, as there are not many prospective studies. In addition, there are varying definitions of OA making it difficult to gather data on the incidence of the disease.[1]
- The most common occupations associated with OA are **bakers, spray painters, health care workers, hairdressers, and cleaners.**[3]

Pathophysiology

There are more than 250 agents that have been identified to cause OA. Table 5-1 is a list of commonly associated allergens causing OA.[4]

TABLE 5-1 AGENTS ASSOCIATED WITH OCCUPATIONAL ASTHMA

Mechanism	Type of agent	Causative agent	Occupations
Immunologic IgE-dependent	HMW agents	Animal urine, dander, serum	Lab workers, veterinarians
		Cereal and soy flour	Bakers, millers
		Enzymes:	
		α-Amylase, cellulase	Bakers, pharmaceutical workers
		Papain, pepsin	Pharmaceutical and food workers
		Bacillus subtilis-derived, *Aspergillus*-derived	Detergent industry workers
		Gums (acacia, guar)	Printers, carpet manufacturers, hairdressers
		Psyllium	Pharmaceutical workers, nurses
		Egg proteins	Egg-processing workers
		Seeds—cottonseed, linseed, flaxseed	Bakers, oil producers
		Storage mites	Farmers, grain store workers
		Latex	Health care workers, manufacturers
Immunologic IgE-dependent (often haptens)	LMW chemicals	Acid anhydrides: Phthalic, trimelitic	Plastic, epoxy resin workers
		Platinum salts	Platinum refinery workers
		Reactive dyes	Textiles and dyeing workers
		Persulfate salts	Hairdressers
Immunologic	LMW chemicals	Diisocyanates: Toluene, methylene diphenyl, hexamethylene	Polyurethane, foundry workers, painters
		Western red cedar-plicatic acid	Sawmill workers, carpenters
		Amines	Photographers, shellac workers, chemist
		Colophony	Electronic workers, welders
Nonimmunologic (toxic effect)	LMW chemicals/irritants	Chlorine	Pulp mill and chemical workers
		Sulfur dioxide	Pyrite workers, miners
		Ammonia	Spray painters, chemical workers
		Sodium fumes	Cleaners, chemical workers
		Smoke	Fire fighters, police officers
		Diisocyanates	Spray painters, polyurethane workers

IgE, immunoglobulin E; HMW, high molecular weight; LMW, low molecular weight.

Sensitizer-induced OA

- HMW sensitizer:
  - Proteins and/or glycoproteins act **as antigens in an immunoglobulin E (IgE)-mediated mechanism**. The allergen occasionally can be well characterized. However, several sensitizers are difficult to identify.[1]
  - This IgE-mediated response leads to **similar pathology seen in nonoccupational asthma (see Chapter 4)**, with bronchial wall thickening, secondary eosinophilic infiltration, smooth muscle hypertrophy, fibroblast proliferation of subepithelium and airway obstruction.
- LMW sensitizer:
  - LMW sensitizers can cause OA by both **IgE and non–IgE-mediated mechanisms**.
  - LMW sensitizers can **haptenate to host proteins and drive IgE expression**.
  - Cell-mediated mechanisms may underlie some immunologic mechanisms to LMW sensitizers.

Irritant-induced OA

- In contrast to sensitizer-induced OA, irritant-induced OA is caused by **direct toxic effects** of these agents on airway tissues (see Table 5-1 for a list of common irritant agents).
- Since these reactions are **not immunologically mediated**, prior exposure is not necessary to induce pathology.
- Exposure to high levels of irritant agents can lead to a cascade of events involving the nonadaptive immunologic response.
- Initially, there is **injury to bronchial epithelial cells** causing release of inflammatory mediators and neurogenic inflammation. Nonspecific macrophage activation occurs with mast cell degranulation.

Risk Factors

- The most important risk factor is the **level and duration of exposure** to agents capable of causing OA. High levels of exposure and long duration of exposure lead to increasing likelihood of occurrence of OA.
- **Atopy** is a risk factor for HMW allergens.
- Patients that develop **occupational rhinitis and/or conjunctivitis** are at increased risk of developing OA.
- There is geographic variation to the incidence of OA. Similar substances in different parts of the world are associated with different rates of OA. This may be due to the variation in exposure, co-exposures, and in recognition of disease.
- **Tobacco smoking.**

Prevention

- Primary prevention efforts should focus on implementing **interventions that reduce exposure** to known OA-causing agents.[4]
- In a facility where there is known sensitizers, new cases of OA can be reduced by limiting ambient exposure to HMW sensitizers and by identifying patients with new occupational allergic symptoms.

DIAGNOSIS

Clinical Presentation

- Patients present with symptoms of asthma including dyspnea, wheezing, chest tightness, and cough.

- Symptoms of rhinitis and conjunctivitis will often precede the development of asthma.
- In OA, these **symptoms should be related to a workplace exposure** to a known OA-causing agent.
- History should include details about **occupational history** and all previous jobs held. The patient should also be asked about the use of **protective equipment**.
- Additional history will help differentiate OA from non–work-related asthma, vocal cord dysfunction, and hypersensitivity pneumonitis.

Differential Diagnosis

In addition to other diseases that can masquerade as asthma, other respiratory diseases should be considered along with OA

- **Hypersensitivity pneumonitis** can usually be distinguished from O.A by radiographic findings, which often show ground-glass nodularities, and pulmonary function testing (PFT) that typically shows restrictive disease.
- **Bronchiolitis obliterans** ("popcorn worker's lung") has been linked to diacetyl exposure in the workplace.

Diagnostic Testing

- Reversible airway limitation should be documented by spirometry and/or bronchial reactivity challenge with histamine, mannitol, or methacholine.
- In addition to establishing the presence of reversible airway obstruction, the diagnosis of OA must be confirmed by the evidence of **work-related symptom worsening**.
- Objective data that can be used to link work place exposure to OA include spirometry, peak flow, and immunologic testing.
- **Serial spirometry or peak expiratory flow rates** (PEFR) are often used to demonstrate a temporal worsening of airway obstruction after workplace exposures.
  ○ This approach is limited by patient compliance, but when used correctly has a high sensitivity and specificity.
  ○ Typically, a patient with suspected OA will record serial flow rates for 2–4 weeks.
  ○ Ideally, the patient will measure PEFR four times daily: Morning, mid-shift, after work, and before sleeping.
  ○ One of those weeks includes a week away from work.
  ○ Patients with OA typically display the following pattern:[1]
    ■ Worsening of peak flow as the day progresses with improvement over the weekend.
    ■ Progressively worsening peak flow as the work week progresses.
    ■ Improvement in peak flows during a week away from work or during vacation.
- **Specific inhalation challenge** can be used to demonstrate reversible airway obstruction after exposure to a specific sensitizer.
  ○ During a specific inhalation challenge, the patient is exposed to a specific sensitizer in a controlled environment.
  ○ This allows the physician to identify a direct causal relationship between a sensitizer and airway obstruction.
  ○ Considered the **gold standard in diagnosis of IgE-mediated OA.**
  ○ Testing is limited by the necessity of trained personnel and emergency equipment.
- **Immunologic testing** can establish sensitization to a particular sensitizer.
  ○ **High negative predictive value**, indicating that if a patient has a negative test to a sensitizer that is a known work-related sensitizer, then the patient likely does not have OA.
  ○ Useful mostly for HMW sensitizers since testing is dependent on IgE-mediated reaction.

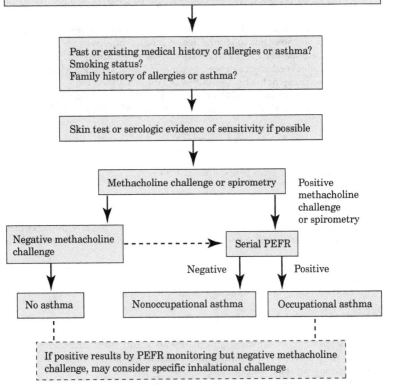

FIGURE 5-1 Algorithm for the diagnosis of occupational asthma. Mean peak expiratory flow rate (PEFR) consistently reduced by <20% with improvement away from work is diagnostic for occupational asthma.

○ Demonstration of sensitization does not necessarily establish that the tested agent is responsible for the patient's respiratory symptoms (specific inhalation challenge may be necessary).
- A simplified diagnostic workflow for OA is presented in Fig. 5-1.

TREATMENT

- The first-line and most important treatment for sensitizer-induced OA is **removal of the patient from the working environment**.
- Pharmacologic treatment of OA is the same as non–work-related asthma. The same treatment guidelines and symptomatic control are applied to the management of OA.
  ○ Pharmacologic treatment is second-line therapy after the removal from the work environment.
  ○ **Patients that continue to be exposed to sensitizer despite optimal medications have poor outcomes due to chronic remodeling of the airways**.
  ○ **Allergen immunotherapy** is a treatment option for sensitized OA. This therapy should only be used when a patient is unable to leave the work environment and when a specific agent has been identified as a cause of OA.[4]
- Patients with irritant-induced OA do not need to be removed from their working environment, but steps should be taken to **prevent further high level of exposure**.

SPECIAL CONSIDERATIONS

- The socioeconomic impact of being diagnosed with OA can have a lasting effect on the patient.
- Continued exposure to offending occupational agent can lead to fatal asthma exacerbation.[4]
- Once a patient has stopped working at the offending work place, many times they have difficulty finding new employment. This can further lead to depression as the patient still has financial obligations.
- In this setting, the specialty physician has a duty to be the patient's advocate in qualifying for disability or workman's compensation.

MONITORING/FOLLOW-UP

- Patients should be monitored approximately on a yearly basis after removal from offending agents. There is evidence that patients may have persistent symptoms even after leaving the work place.[4]
- If patients are unable to leave the work place, more frequent monitoring may be indicated based on the severity of symptoms.[4]

OUTCOME/PROGNOSIS

- Outcomes of patients with OA depend on the removal of exposure to offending agent, duration of exposure, and severity of symptoms during exposure.[5]
- If the patient is no longer exposed to the offending agent, the prognosis is excellent.

REFERENCES

1. Dykewicz M. Occupational asthma: current concepts in pathogenesis, diagnosis and management. *J Allergy Clin Immunol.* 2009;123:519–528.
2. Bernstein IL, Chang-Yeung M, Malo J-L, et al., eds. *Asthma in the Work-Place.* New York, NY: Marcel Dekkar, 1993.
3. Smith A, Berstein D. Management of work-related Asthma. *J Allergy Clin Immunol.* 2009;123: 551–577.
4. Malo JL, Chang-Yeung M. Agents causing occupational asthma. *J Allergy Clin Immunol.* 2009;123:545–550.
5. Masetrelli P, Boscheto P, Fabbri L, et al. Mechanisms of occupational asthma. *J Allergy Clin Immunol.* 2009;123:531.

Hypersensitivity Pneumonitis

6

Olajumoke O. Fadugba

GENERAL PRINCIPLES

Definition

- Hypersensitivity pneumonitis (HP), previously called extrinsic allergic alveolitis, is a disease caused by **inappropriate immunologic reaction to inhaled antigens,** resulting in respiratory and systemic symptoms.
- Diagnosis is based on a history of antigen exposure, clinical features, radiographic, laboratory, physiologic, and sometimes histopathologic findings. It is a complex syndrome of varying intensity and natural history and may mimic other chronic lung diseases such as sarcoidosis and idiopathic pulmonary fibrosis (IPF).

Classification

- Clinical presentation is classically characterized as acute, subacute, and chronic depending on the intensity, frequency and duration of exposure, and the severity of the host's immune inflammatory response.
- The three forms of the syndrome are not stages of a single disease process, as patients with acute HP do not necessarily progress to chronic disease, and patients who present with the chronic form may not have the acute presentation.[1]

Epidemiology

- The greatest risk factor for developing HP is **exposure to inhaled organic particles and chemical compounds.** Contact with birds (e.g., pigeons, parakeets), humidifiers, moldy wood, and other environmental settings can increase risk (Table 6-1).[2]
  - Farmer's lung was the first form of HP described in farmers of the early 20th century exposed to moldy straw and hay.
  - **Genetic factors** have also been postulated to contribute to risk.
  - Cigarette smoking may decrease the risk of HP in exposed individuals.[3]
- The incidence of HP varies depending on location, season, local practices, and host response.
- Estimates of the true prevalence and incidence of HP are largely unknown because HP is rare, the lack of consistent clinical definition for HP, and the few cohort studies on the incidence or prevalence of the disease.

Etiology

- There is a wide range of occupations and inhaled agents that can cause HP (Table 6-1).[2]
- **Most antigens are organic,** but some low molecular weight chemical compounds can form haptens with serum albumin to create an antigenic particle.[3]
- Inhaled particles must be small enough (<5 μm) to reach the lung parenchyma and trigger an immune response.

TABLE 6-1	EXAMPLES OF ETIOLOGIC AGENTS IN HYPERSENSITIVITY PNEUMONITIS	
Disease	**Environmental source**	**Antigen**
Farmer's lung	Moldy hay and grain	Thermophilic actinomycetes, e.g., *Saccharopolyspora rectivirgula*
Bird fancier's lung	Pigeons, parakeets	Avian serum, droppings, and feather proteins
Bagassosis	Moldy sugar cane	*Thermoactinomyces sacchari, Tylenchorhynchus vulgaris*
Wine maker's lung	Moldy grapes	*Botrytis cinerea*
Coffee worker's lung	Coffee bean dust	Unknown
Tobacco grower's lung	Tobacco plants	*Aspergillus* species
Humidifier fever	Humidifier reservoirs, air conditioners, aquaria	Thermophilic actinomycetes, *Klebsiella oxytoca, Naegleria gruberi, Acanthamoeba* species
Hot tub lung	Mist, moldy ceilings, and tubs	*Mycobacterium avium* complex, *Cladosporium* species
Laboratory worker's lung	Laboratory rats	Rat serum, pelts, and urine proteins
Malt worker's disease	Moldy barley	*Aspergillus clavatus, A. fumigatus*
Wood dust pneumonitis	Oak, cedar, mahogany, pine dust	*Alternaria* species, *Bacillus subtilis*
Chemical worker's lung		Diphenylmethane diisocyanate, toluene diisocyanate, and others

Adapted from: Hirschmann JV, Pipavath SN, Godwin JD. Hypersensitivity pneumonitis: a historical, clinical, and radiologic review. *Radiographics* 2009;29:1921–1938.

- The causative agents for HP continue to increase as societal practices change.
  - Household mold has been increasingly implicated in causing HP.
  - Over the past decade, the incidence of humidifier lung has increased, while farmer's lung incidence has decreased.[4]

Pathophysiology

- HP is an immune-mediated disease with possible roles for both antibody and cellular immune responses.
  - The immune response to the inciting antigen can cause **expression of antibodies** resulting in immune complex formation (type III hypersensitivity).
    - High titer, antigen-specific, precipitating serum antibody to the inciting antigen can result in complement fixation.
    - Presence of precipitating antibodies to specific antigen is an important diagnostic markers of HP.

○ **Cell-mediated mechanisms** (type IV hypersensitivity) are also likely to be contributing to disease.
  ▪ Fixation of complement results in the recruitment of inflammatory cells including lymphocytes and macrophages.
  ▪ Once present in the lung tissue, these immune cells are thought to secrete Th1 skewed cytokines, including interferon gamma, which promotes persistent inflammation and granuloma formation.
- Genetics may also influence the development of HP. Polymorphisms in tumor necrosis factor (TNF)-α and HLA haplotypes have been implicated in pathogenesis.
- Acute HP is characterized by a neutrophilic infiltrate, which is later replaced by activated lymphocytes with a predominance of CD8+ over CD4+ cells.
- Subacute HP demonstrates non-caseating granulomas (demonstrating less organization than in sarcoidosis).
- Chronic HP may or may not show granulomas but demonstrates interstitial fibrosis, particularly in the upper lobes of the lung.

Prevention

- HP can be prevented by reducing exposure to causative agents and using protective equipment.
- **Antigen reduction** focuses on ridding environments of antigenic particles:
  ○ Wetting compost before handling reduces dispersion of actinomycete spores.
  ○ Using antimicrobial agents while processing sugar cane reduces mold growth.
- **Facility design** can reduce the chances of contamination of the work environment:
  ○ Moisture plays a large role in indoor microbial overgrowth.
  ○ Humidity in buildings should be kept below 60%, carpeting should be avoided in moist areas, and water in ventilating systems should not be recirculated.
- **Protective devices:** In circumstances where it is impossible to completely eliminate environmental antigens, controls such as respirators should be used.[5]

DIAGNOSIS

Clinical Presentation

- Despite the diversity of inhaled agents that can cause HP, that there are various diseases present with similar symptoms, suggesting that they share pathogenic features.
- Affected patients present with interstitial pneumonitis in one of the three forms of the disease:
  ○ **Acute HP:** This form usually occurs within 4–6 hours of exposure. It is the most easily recognized form and presents with **fever, chills, malaise, cough, and dyspnea without wheezing.** Symptoms last for hours to days and can be confused with viral or bacterial illness. Physical examination often reveals tachypnea and fine inspiratory crackles especially at the lung bases; wheezing is rarely heard.
  ○ **Subacute HP:** This is characterized by **more gradual onset of low-grade fever, cough, progressive dyspnea, fatigue, and sometimes anorexia and weight loss.** This may be superimposed with acute episodes. Examination reveals tachypnea, lung crackles, and sometimes cyanosis. This, like acute HP, is usually reversible with the removal of antigen.

○ **Chronic HP:** This form often occurs with exposure to antigen for a long period. It presents with **insidious onset** over a period of months to years, with **progressive cough, dyspnea, fatigue, and weight loss.** Examination may reveal cyanosis and if digital clubbing is seen, suggests poor prognosis. This form is often disabling and is **usually irreversible.**[3]

Differential Diagnosis

There are many diseases apart from HP that are associated with inhalation of organic agents. Furthermore, other syndromes have clinical or histologic features similar to HP.

- **Inhalation fever** (e.g., metal fume fever): Occurs a few hours after inhaling the substance; characterized by fever, malaise, myalgias, headache, without significant pulmonary symptoms. This is self-limited (usually within 24 hours) without long-term effects.[6]
- **Organic dust toxic syndrome** (ODTS): This, unlike HP, is a **nonimmunologic** reaction to inhaled antigens. It is **much more common in farmers than HP** and is caused by exposure to **mycotoxins** or **endotoxins** produced by fungi found in moldy hay, grains, and *Fusarium*-contaminated textile materials. Symptoms and findings include fever, myalgias, cough, dyspnea 4–6 hours post-exposure, leukocytosis, and normal lung function or mild restriction with reduced diffusion capacity of carbon monoxide (DLCO). Notably with ODTS, serum precipitins are negative and there are no long-term sequelae.[7]
- Chronic bronchitis: This is **much more common than HP in farmers.** The immune mechanism of HP and chronic obstructive pulmonary disease in nonsmokers is thought to be related.
- **Sarcoidosis:** Both HP and sarcoidosis have lymphocytosis on bronchoalveolar lavage (BAL) and may demonstrate noncaseating granulomas on lung biopsy. However, granulomas in sarcoidosis have distribution in bronchial wall and perivascular locations while HP granulomas have a centrilobular distribution. Also in sarcoidosis, there is less lymphocytosis (around 50% vs. 70% in HP), with a predominance of CD4+ cells as opposed to CD8+ T-cell predominance in HP, though this distinction has recently been challenged.[3]
- IPF: The chronic form of HP can be distinguished from IPF partly by findings of centrilobular opacities and lack of lower lobe-predominant fibrosis in HP.[2]

Diagnostic Testing

- Diagnosis of HP is based on history of exposure, clinical picture, imaging, and physiologic findings.
- Other testing may be useful in solidifying the diagnosis of HP or ruling out other potential diseases.
- Identifying the causative agent is particularly important to prevent ongoing exposure.

Laboratories

- **Serum precipitins:** Most patients with HP have precipitating immunoglobulin G (IgG) antibodies specific to the inhaled antigen.
  ○ These antibodies are often present in asymptomatic exposed people as well; only 1–15% of people exposed to an offending antigen develop the disease. Therefore, **the presence of serum precipitins simply indicates exposure** and not necessarily disease.

- ○ Absence of serum precipitins **does not rule out HP** because some HP-associated antigens may not be present in the routine precipitin panel and some antigens are still undiscovered.
- ○ There are several methods for detecting precipitins. The conventional Ouchterlony double immunodiffusion test is limited in both sensitivity and specificity. **Enzyme-linked immunosorbent assay (ELISA)** is a preferred method, but also lacks standardization.[1,3]
- Other laboratory tests:
  - ○ Nonspecific laboratories such as erythrocyte sedimentation rate (ESR), C-reactive protein (CRP), rheumatoid factor (RF), and lactate dehydrogenase (LDH) may be elevated in HP.
  - ○ Serum IgE and eosinophils are not typically elevated.
  - ○ **Skin tests are not useful** in the diagnosis of HP.

Imaging
- **Chest radiographs** in patients with HP may be normal or show discrete nodules or diffuse, poorly defined infiltrates in the acute or subacute form of the disease. Chronic HP may show reticulonodular infiltrates, fibrosis, or honeycombing.
- **High resolution CT** (HRCT) in being increasingly used to aid the diagnosis of HP.
  - ○ Various changes can be seen including honeycombing, and fibrosis, especially in chronic HP.
  - ○ **Centrilobular ground-glass opacities are a differentiating feature of HP.**
  - ○ Additionally, pathologic changes in HP can demonstrate a characteristic distribution:
    - ■ **Acute HP shows abnormalities more prominent in the lower lung zones while chronic disease is manifested more in the upper zones of the lung.**
    - ■ Most inhaled antigens deposit in the dependent (lower) lung regions.
    - ■ Lymphatic clearance of antigens in the upper zones is slower than that in the lower zones of the lung. Therefore, with chronic antigen exposure, the upper lung zones are more severely damaged.
  - ○ Findings not usually associated with HP are lung cavities, hilar adenopathy, and pleural thickening.[1]

Diagnostic Procedures

Inhalation Challenge
- Inhalation challenge can be used to link HP symptoms to the suspected antigen.
- A patient can be exposed to the offending environment, after which symptoms are observed. Alternatively, in a controlled environment (such as a hospital), the patient is exposed to the suspected antigen via a nebulizer.
- Changes in clinical picture, pulmonary function tests (PFTs), and chest imaging are studied for 24 hours.
- These tests are limited in utility as the **inhalation protocols lack standardization**.[3]

Pulmonary Function Testing
- PFTs cannot distinguish HP from other interstitial lung disease.
- PFTs are used to measure functional impairment and can help guide treatment (e.g., who should get corticosteroid treatment).
- **Characteristically, PFTs show a restrictive pattern with decreased DLCO.**
- An obstructive pattern can predominate in more insidious forms of HP, especially as emphysematous changes develop.
- Mixed restrictive and obstructive defects can also occur.

Bronchoalveolar Lavage

- BAL is an important tool in supporting the diagnosis of HP.
- **Neutrophils in BAL fluid increase early after antigen exposure.**
- **The BAL fluid in the subacute and chronic forms of HP has marked lymphocytosis,** with the percentage of lymphocytes ranging between 60 and 70% (normal is 6–8%).
- HP typically demonstrates more CD8+ than CD4+ T cells with a CD4+/CD8+ T-cell ratio of less than 1. This is in contrast to the BAL fluid in sarcoidosis where CD4+/CD8+ ratio is usually 5:1 or greater.
- Eosinophils are not increased (except in some advanced cases), but mast cells and basophils can be increased.[1,3]
- A normal BAL lymphocyte count essentially rules out active disease.

Lung Biopsy

- Lung biopsy is sometimes needed to confirm the diagnosis of HP and can be obtained by transbronchial means or surgically.
- Lung biopsy should be reserved for patients with a very unusual presentation or unexpected response to treatment, given the possible morbidity associated with surgical biopsy.
- Histopathologic findings include **interstitial lymphocyte and plasma cell infiltrates, small, poorly formed noncaseating granulomas, and macrophages with foamy cytoplasm in the alveoli.**
- In chronic stages, peribronchiolar fibrosis can be seen. Schaumann bodies (calcium and protein inclusions) within isolated Langhans giant cells can also be seen.[3]

TREATMENT

- The principles of HP management are twofold: **Avoidance of antigen exposure and glucocorticoids.**
- Avoidance of the offending antigen through environmental control is the cornerstone of therapy in HP.
- If antigen exposure is related to the patient's job, avoidance can be difficult because of the potential loss of livelihood.
- Antigen can often persist at home despite removal of the primary offending agent (e.g., birds). In such cases, professional control measures and environmental modification may be sought.

Medications

- Some patients benefit from corticosteroids, the only drugs currently used for HP.
- Indications for use are acute, severe, or progressive disease.
- Glucocorticoids help to control symptoms but do not improve long-term outcome.
- The recommended regimen is 40–60 mg of prednisone or its equivalent corticosteroid. Treatment duration is 1–2 weeks followed by a taper over 2–4 weeks.[3,8,9]

OUTCOME/PROGNOSIS

- **The majority of patients with HP recover fully after they are removed from the offending environment,** and some recover despite continued exposure.
- Among the most well-studied types of HP, bird fancier's lung has a worse prognosis than famer's lung.

- **Patients with chronic HP who have fibrosis or honeycombing on HRCT or lung biopsy clearly have worse prognosis,** and their disease may be irreversible despite environmental control or corticosteroid therapy.
- **The risk of mortality increases with lower DLCO, oxygen desaturation following exercise (≤88%), and more severe restrictive ventilatory defects on PFTs.**

REFERENCES

1. Knutsen AP, Amin RS, Temprano J, et al. Hypersensitivity pneumonitis and eosinophilic pulmonary diseases. In: Victor C, Kendig E, eds. *Kendig's Disorders of the Respiratory Tract in Children,* 7th ed. Philadelphia, PA: Saunders/Elsevier, 2006:686–693.
2. Hirschmann JV, Pipavath SN, Godwin JD. Hypersensitivity pneumonitis: a historical, clinical, and radiologic review. *Radiographics* 2009;29:1921–1938.
3. Girard M, Lacasse Y, Cormier Y. Hypersensitivity pneumonitis. *Allergy* 2009;64:322–334.
4. Girard M, Cormier Y. Hypersensitivity pneumonitis.*Curr Opin Allergy Clin Immunol* 2010; 10:99–103.
5. Dion G, Duchaine A, Meriaux A, et al. Hypersensitivity pneumonitis (HP) prevention: benefits of industry and research community collaboration. *Am J Respir Crit Care Med* 2008; 177:A555.
6. Kaye P, Young H, O'Sullivan I. Metal fume fever: a case report and review of the literature. *Emerg Med J* 2002;19:268–269.
7. Seifert SA, Von Essen S, Jacobitz K, et al. Organic dust toxic syndrome: a review. *J Toxicol Clin Toxicol* 2003;41:185–193.
8. Mönkäre S. Influence of corticosteroid treatment on the course of farmer's lung. *Eur J Respir Dis* 1983;64:283–293.
9. Kokkarinen JI, Tukiainen HO, Terho EO. Effect of corticosteroid treatment on the recovery of pulmonary function in farmer's lung. *Am Rev Respir Dis* 1992;145:3–5.

Pulmonary Function Tests

Ashley Emmert

GENERAL PRINCIPLES

Definition

- Pulmonary function tests (PFTs) include several different methods of assessing the functional characteristics of an individual's lungs. As such, they are valuable adjuncts to the treatment and assessment of respiratory diseases.
- Common PFTs utilized in clinical practice include spirometry, lung volume measurement, and the diffusion capacity.

Classification

- **Spirometry** is a PFT that measures the dynamic airflow during the respiratory cycle.
  - Commonly used abbreviations and values derived from PFTs are shown in Table 7-1.
  - **Flow volume loops** can be invaluable in difficult diagnostic cases by providing insight into functional characteristics of upper and lower airways as well as possible functional defects due to extrathoracic causes.
- **Lung volume** PFTs measure the absolute capacity of a patient's lungs.
- **Diffusion capacity** measurement is a type of PFT that measures the ability of the lung to transport gasses.

DIAGNOSIS

- PFTs are obtained for various reasons.
- Diagnosis:
  - Evaluate presence of pulmonary disease.
  - Evaluate symptoms of dyspnea, cough, or wheezing.
  - Screen for high-risk individuals (e.g., smokers or those with occupational exposures).
  - Pre-operative evaluation.
- Monitoring:
  - Assess response to bronchodilator therapy.
  - Follow progression of present pulmonary disease.
  - Assess for adverse reactions to drugs that may have pulmonary side effects (e.g., amiodarone).
  - Assess pulmonary dysfunction in response to environmental exposures.
- Other:
  - Documentation of disability for insurance.
  - Assess for qualifications for rehabilitation programs.

TABLE 7-1	ABBREVIATIONS USED IN PULMONARY FUNCTION TESTING	
Measurement	Abbreviation	Description
Forced vital capacity	FVC	The volume of gas that can be forcefully expelled after maximal inhalation
Forced expiratory volume in 1 second	FEV_1	The volume measured in the first second of maximal forced exhalation
Forced expiratory flow during 25–75% of vital capacity	$FEF_{25-75\%}$	The maximal mid-expiratory flow rate
Peak expiratory flow	PEF	The maximal airflow rate achieved during expiration
Total lung capacity	TLC	The volume of lungs after maximal inspiration
Vital capacity	VC	The volume of gas measured with slow expiration after maximal inhalation
Functional residual capacity	FRC	The volume left in lungs after normal exhalation (TLC–inspiratory capacity)
Arterial blood gas	ABG	
Diffusion capacity of lung for carbon monoxide (CO)	DLCO	The diffusion capacity between capillary and alveolar wall using CO

- Follow-up spirograms are used mainly for monitoring purposes and can be repeated at the physician's discretion. For asthma patients, guidelines recommend an initial diagnostic spirogram and at least one annually for the management of therapy.

Diagnostic Testing

- Spirometry is generally performed by one of two methods:
  - Open-circuit spirometry is generally cheaper to perform.
  - Closed-circuit spirometry allows more accurate measurement of the functional residual capacity (FRC), but because the patient breathes into the machine, maintaining good hygiene is a concern.
  - Normal baseline values for spirometry are dependent on various factors including sex, age, weight, and height.
  - Spirometry is a **patient effort–dependent** test that requires the understanding and cooperation of patients for accurate and reproducible test results.
    - The minimum number of respiratory loops needed is three, and the best forced expiratory volume in 1 second (FEV_1) and forced vital capacity (FVC) of the three test values should be recorded and used for interpretation.
    - The maximum recommended number for consecutive testing is eight, because patient fatigue becomes a significant factor after more than eight trials.

○ **Criteria for acceptable spirometry** from the American Thoracic Society include[1]:
  ■ A smooth continuous exhalation for >6 seconds demonstrating a plateau, defined as no change in the volume for at least 1 second during expiration.
  ■ A satisfactory start of test without hesitation or false start.
  ■ Lack of artifacts such as coughing, glottic closure, early termination of exhalation, or obstructed mouth piece.
  ■ Properly calibrated equipment without leak.
○ The reproducibility of lung function tests are important not only for following the longitudinal trends but also to ensure that such tests can be compared from one test center to the another. **Criteria for reproducibility** include[1]:
  ■ The largest FVC should be within 0.15 L of the second largest FVC value.
  ■ The largest FEV_1 should be within 0.15 L of the second largest FEV_1.
  ■ Additional spirograms (maximum of eight) should be obtained to assure that the above criteria are met in at least three of the maneuvers.
○ An algorithm for interpretation of PFTs is shown in Fig. 7-1.

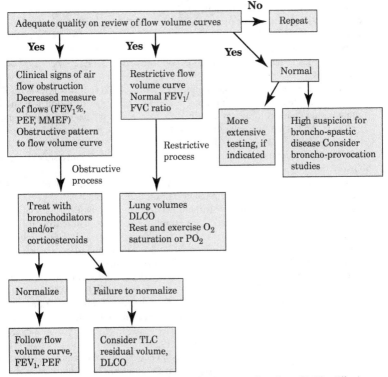

FIGURE 7-1 Algorithm for interpretation of pulmonary function. DLCO, diffusion capacity of lung for carbon monoxide; FEV_1, forced expiratory volume in 1 second; FVC, forced vital capacity; MMEF, maximal mid expiratory flow; PEF, peak expiratory flow; PO_2, partial pressure of oxygen; TLC, total lung capacity.

TABLE 7-2	SAMPLE PULMONARY FUNCTION TESTS OF A PATIENT WITH ASTHMA				
	Before bronchodilator		After bronchodilator		
	Actual	% predicted	Actual	% predicted	% change
FVC (L)	3.14	67	4.32	92	25
FEV$_1$ (L)	2.12	53	3.24	81	28
FEV$_1$:FVC (%)		67		75	
FEF$_{25-75\%}$ (L/sec)	0.63	14	1.43	33	
TLC (L)	6.45	100			
DLCO (mL/min/ mm Hg)	32	100			

- Evidence of **airway obstruction** can be made with PFTs.
  - ○ When airway obstruction is present, the values of FEV$_1$ and FVC can both be reduced, but FEV$_1$ is disproportionately reduced compared to FVC, thus giving a **lower FEV$_1$:FVC ratio.**
    - ■ The primary criterion for the diagnosis of obstruction is FEV$_1$:FVC <87% of predicted.
    - ■ Occasionally, in the face of borderline FEV$_1$:FVC, earlier airflow obstruction may be detected by forced expiratory flow (FEF) 25–75%, the rationale being that earlier changes in airway obstruction start in the smaller and peripheral airways. This is a nonspecific finding and should not be used as a criterion for the diagnosis of small airways disease.
  - ○ In **asthma,** the primary functional abnormality is the presence of reversible airway obstruction.
    - ■ This can be demonstrated on spirometry by the measurement of FEV$_1$ and FVC before and after the administration of bronchodilators.
    - ■ **Reversibility of >12% of FEV$_1$** (or 200 mL increase from baseline) supports a diagnosis of asthma. See Table 7-2 for sample PFTs of a patient with asthma.
    - ■ The absence of improvement after bronchodilator treatment does not exclude reversible obstruction. Obstruction may be due to inflammation, which may only be reversible after prolonged antiinflammatory therapy.
  - ○ In chronic obstructive pulmonary disease **(COPD)/emphysema,** there is an obstructive pattern of PFTs with reduction in the ratio of FEV$_1$:FVC, but this obstruction is **usually not responsive to bronchodilator administration.** See Table 7-3 for sample PFTs of a patient with emphysema/COPD.
    - ■ In contrast to asthma, the diffusion capacity of the lung for carbon monoxide (DLCO) is often reduced in COPD.
    - ■ In advanced disease air trapping becomes more evident—the total lung capacity (TLC) and residual volume (RV) increase, resulting in an increase in the RV:TLC ratio.
  - ○ **Restrictive lung disease** is characterized by a decreased **TLC <70% of predicted.**
    - ■ FEV$_1$ and FVC are usually proportionately reduced and, therefore, will give a normal ratio of FEV$_1$:FVC.

| TABLE 7-3 | SAMPLE PULMONARY FUNCTION TESTS OF A PATIENT WITH EMPHYSEMA/CHRONIC OBSTRUCTIVE PULMONARY DISEASE |

	Before bronchodilator		After bronchodilator		
	Actual	% predicted	Actual	% predicted	% change
FVC (L)	2.5	62	2.5	62	0
FEV_1 (L)	1.58	50	1.44	46	−4
FEV_1:FVC (%)		63		57	
$FEF_{25-75\%}$ (L/sec)	1.3	33	1.3	33	
RV (L)	4	160			
TLC (L)	7.12	110			
D_{LCO} (mL/min/ mm Hg)	25	78			

- As the disease process progresses FVC may decrease faster than FEV_1 and, thus, can increase the ratio. See Table 7-4 for sample PFTs of a patient with restrictive lung disease.
- Restrictive defects are graded based on the severity of decrease in TLC or vital capacity (VC).
- **Peak expiratory flow rates** (PEFRs) can be calculated from a spirogram or measured with a hand-held peak flow meter.
  - Peak expiratory flows can be used to roughly diagnose asthma; however, this is not a recommended practice.
  - The PEFR is used as an outpatient tool in measuring response to therapy as well as monitoring early symptoms of exacerbation or helping to identify provocative factors.
  - Normal values of PEFR are based on age, gender, and height.
    - In addition, there is a well-documented **diurnal variation** to the peak flow values, with lowest values occurring in the early morning on awakening and highest values obtained during 4–6 p.m.
    - It is important to obtain values in the mornings and the evenings. Each measurement should be the highest value from three consecutive maneuvers.

| TABLE 7-4 | SAMPLE PULMONARY FUNCTION TESTS OF A PATIENT WITH RESTRICTIVE LUNG DISEASE |

	Actual	% predicted
FVC (L)	1.8	45
FEV_1 (L)	1.62	47
FEV_1:FVC (%)	90	
$FEF_{25-75\%}$ (L/sec)	1.4	41
TLC (L)	4.16	65

- If there is 20% diurnal variation, this is a suggestion of airway hyperresponsiveness and further treatment or testing should be instituted.
  - Adult patients are able to correctly identify symptom exacerbations before a decrease in the peak flow meter values. However, pediatric patients and their parents report being symptom free until the peak expiratory flow values are in the worrisome range.
  - Peak flow meters provide some valuable objective measurements to follow and tailor therapy. Alert values are usually divided into three zones: Green, yellow, and red.
    - Green: No symptoms (>80% of baseline maximal PEFR).
    - Yellow: Mild symptoms (50–80% of baseline maximal PEFR).
    - Red: Moderate to severe symptoms (<50% of baseline PEFR).
  - PEFR <80% of baseline usually signals need for contacting a physician and possible escalation of treatment, either with an increasing dose/frequency of β-agonist, a course of antibiotics, adjustment of other medications, or a course of oral corticosteroids.
- Bronchial hyperresponsiveness (BHR) can be documented via **bronchoprovocation** with agents known to cause bronchial constriction.[2]
  - BHR is a hallmark feature of asthma that is demonstrable in nearly all patients with asthma.
  - Bronchoprovocation challenges are performed for:
    - Suspicion of asthma by history but nondiagnostic PFTs.
    - Assessing the relative risk for developing occupational asthma.
    - Evaluation of severity of occupational asthma.
  - **Absolute contraindications** for bronchoprovocation challenge are:
    - Severe airflow obstruction (FEV_1 <50% predicted or <1 L).
    - Myocardial infarction or stroke within 3 months.
    - Uncontrolled hypertension with systolic blood pressure >200 or diastolic blood pressure >100.
    - Known aortic aneurysm.
  - Relative contraindications include:
    - Moderate airflow obstruction (FEV_1 <60% predicted or <1.5 L).
    - Inability to cooperate or follow directions for test.
    - Current use of cholinesterase inhibitor medication.
    - Pregnancy or breastfeeding (methacholine is considered category C in pregnancy).
  - Medications that can decrease bronchial responsiveness are presented in Table 7-5.
  - Methacholine, histamine, and mannitol challenges are commonly used methods of testing BHR.
    - **Methacholine is the agent of choice** among many clinicians because of the extensive clinical experience and reduced side effects.
    - Histamine challenges can have systemic side effects, such as headache, tachycardia, and flushing. Another disadvantage to histamine is that tachyphylaxis can develop at higher concentrations and with consecutive repeated exposures.
    - Mannitol challenge is a newer pharmacologic agent used to test for BHR that is thought to induce hyperresponsiveness by changing the osmolarity of the bronchial epithelial surface, resulting in mast cell degranulation.
  - There are two methods for performing bronchoprovocation challenge:
    - In the **2-minute tidal breathing protocol**, the patient is given increasing doses of bronchoprovocation agent via nebulizer and should breathe tidal breaths for

TABLE 7-5	MEDICATIONS TO WITHHOLD BEFORE BRONCHOPROVOCATION TESTING	
Medication		**Minimum hold time (hours)**
Short-acting β-agonists:		
Albuterol		8
Intermediate-acting anticholinergics:		
Ipratropium		24
Long-acting β-agonists:		
Salmeterol		48
Formoterol		48
Long-acting anticholinergics:		
Tiotropium		48
Oral bronchodilators:		
Short-acting theophyllines		12
Intermediate-acting theophyllines		24
Long-acting theophyllines		48
Standard β-agonist		12
Long-acting β-agonist		24
Mast cell stabilizers:		
Cromolyn sodium		8
Nedocromil		48
Antihistamines:		
Hydroxyzine		72
Cetirizine		72
Leukotriene modifiers		24
Caffeine		Day of study

Adapted from: Crapo RO, Casaburi R, Coates AL, et al. Guidelines for methacholine and exercise challenge testing-1999. *Am J Respir Crit Care Med* 2000;161:309–329.

exactly 2 minutes. FEV_1 is measured at the end of each 2 minutes and the highest FEV_1 from the acceptable volume loops is recorded. If the FEV_1 changes by <20% from the baseline, then the next dose is given. However, if the FEV_1 changes by >20% from baseline, then the test is terminated, and patient should be assessed for symptoms. At the conclusion of the test, inhaled albuterol is administered, and after 10 minutes, repeat spirometry is obtained.

- In the **five-breath dosimeter protocol,** the patient is given a nebulizer with dosimeter attached, and doses of bronchoprovocation agent are administered after complete exhalation. The patient takes slow (5 seconds), deep breaths through the mouthpiece for a total of five breaths, which should be completed in 2 minutes. FEV_1 is measured approximately 30 seconds and 90 seconds after the fifth inhalation. These maneuvers are repeated until FEV_1 decreases by >20% or the maximal concentration is reached. Once the test is terminated, inhaled albuterol is administered and spirometry is repeated 10 minutes later.

○ **Measurement of response** to the bronchial challenge can be expressed in various ways.

- Common methods include reporting the changes in FEV_1, airways resistance, maximum expiratory flow volume curves, or total respiratory resistance.

- The most widely used method in clinical practice is the **measurement of decrease in FEV$_1$.** This is reported in conjunction with the **provocative concentration 20** (PC20), which is defined as the concentration of constrictor agent at which FEV$_1$ falls by 20% from baseline.
- **Positive test results** (for methacholine) are usually defined as a PC20 <8 mg/mL or 16 mg/mL. Methacholine is a nonspecific bronchoconstrictor and can lead to bronchoconstriction in all people when given in high enough doses. Whether the patient should be diagnosed with asthma requires critical assessment of the pretest probability and clinical suspicion. **Asthmatic patients usually have a positive response at concentrations lower than 8 mg/mL.**
- A **negative test result** (for methacholine) is defined as the absence of bronchial constriction at concentration >16 mg/mL. **A negative test has a higher predictive value and rules out the diagnosis of asthma.**

REFERENCES

1. Miller MR, Hankinson J, Brusasco V, et al. Standardisation of spirometry. *Eur Respir J* 2005;26:319–338.
2. Crapo RO, Casaburi R, Coates AL, et al. Guidelines for methacholine and exercise challenge testing-1999. *Am J Respir Crit Care Med* 2000;161:309–329.

In Vivo and *In Vitro* Diagnostic Tests of Allergy

8

Seth M. Hollander

GENERAL PRINCIPLES

- Many clinical tests have been created to help detect specific antigen sensitivities.
- The most commonly used tests detect the presence of immunoglobulin E (IgE) antibodies against known antigens and include skin testing and *in vitro* measurements of IgE.
- While testing can be very useful, it is not a substitute for a thorough history as sensitization, that is, the presence of specific IgE antibody, is not the same as allergy, which is sensitization leading to clinically observed symptoms.

DIAGNOSIS

Immediate Hypersensitivity Skin Testing

- Immediate hypersensitivity skin testing is an *in vivo* measure of the presence of an **antigen-specific IgE.**
- This is the most sensitive and cost-effective method to screen existing IgE sensitivities that may be responsible for clinical symptoms.
- The antigen is applied to the skin surface by different methods including epicutaneous and intradermal methods.
- The response recorded is due to immediate hypersensitivity and manifests as a **"wheal and flair" reaction.**
  - The wheal is the area of swelling and edema surrounding the site of allergen exposure.
  - The flair refers to the erythema around a site of allergen exposure resulting from vasodilation.
  - Both are measured when assessing the allergic response through skin testing.
- Skin testing **should be performed by a trained professional who is familiar with possible adverse reactions** and the implications of a positive or a negative test result as it relates to the patient's symptom history and clinical picture.

Indications
- Documentation of allergic sensitivity to the specific allergens in patients with the following conditions[1]:
  - Asthma (both to aeroallergens and occupational allergens)
  - Rhinitis
  - Conjunctivitis
  - Food allergy
  - Certain drug allergies

○ Insect hypersensitivity
○ Allergic bronchopulmonary aspergillosis
○ Local anesthetics
- Skin testing is needed for choosing allergen immunotherapy extracts.

Epicutaneous Skin Tests

- These methods introduce the antigen into the epidermis of the skin and thereby activate any IgE-sensitized mast cells by the cross-linking of IgE molecules present on the mast cell surface.
- This, in turn, releases mediators from the mast cell, including histamine, tryptase, chymase, and heparin.
- Typically, the local reaction will be detectable by wheal-and-flare reaction within 15 minutes. However, some sensitivities are not detectable by this method, and further testing (i.e., intradermal skin tests, see later) is needed.[1]
- Preferred areas for testing are the back and volar aspect of the arm.
- Epicutaneous skin tests include prick and puncture techniques.
  ○ **Prick skin testing**[2]:
    ■ The prick skin test is performed by placing a small drop of allergen on the cleansed skin surface and passing a 25- or 26-gauge needle through the antigen at a 45-degree angle.
    ■ The needle should be lightly pressed into the epidermis and then lifted, creating a break in the epidermis without causing bleeding.
    ■ Test antigens should be placed >2 cm from one another.
    ■ Various hollow and solid bore needles and blood lancets are available under different trade names.
  ○ **Puncture skin testing**[2]:
    ■ The puncture skin test is performed by placing a small drop of the allergen extract on the cleansed skin surface and then puncturing the skin with a device at a perpendicular angle, penetrating 1–1.5 mm into the skin.
    ■ Disposable commercially available devices made of plastic allow for placement of multiple antigen test sites at one time.
    ■ Each test antigen site should be placed >2 cm apart.

Intradermal Skin Testing

- Intradermal skin testing is **more sensitive than the epicutaneous skin tests, but it is generally only performed if the epicutaneous test is negative.**[1]
- The test is performed using 25- to 27-gauge needles. A small amount of allergen extract (0.02–0.05 mL; 0.02 mL in hymenoptera to avoid false-positive) is injected intracutaneously, creating a small bleb 2–3 mm in diameter.[2]
- Spaces between each injection site should be >2 cm.
- For patients with a negative prick–puncture test, the concentration of extract for intradermal testing should be between 100- and 1,000-fold more dilute than the concentration used for epicutaneous testing.[1,2]
- **Variability in test results** is often due to common errors, which include injecting too deeply, using too much extract, or causing bleeding. Injecting the extract too deeply may hide the response, thereby giving a false-negative result. On the other hand, use of too much extract or bleeding from the prick or puncture may give false-positive results.[2]

Test Controls
- Positive controls[2]:
  - ○ **Histamine** at 1 mg/mL for epicutaneous methods and 0.1 mg/mL for intradermal skin testing is used.
  - ○ A patient must have a positive response to the histamine control to proceed with the skin testing.
    - ■ Lack of an appropriate response to a positive control invalidates skin testing results.
    - ■ Possible causes of a negative response to a histamine control include medications (see later) and certain skin conditions.
  - ○ Mast cell degranulators, such as codeine or morphine sulfate, may also be used as positive controls.
- Negative controls[2]:
  - ○ **Diluents** used to preserve the allergen extracts are used as negative controls.
  - ○ This will help detect any problems with technique, possible skin irritation reaction, or dermatographism.

Interpretation of Skin Test Results
- The immediate hypersensitivity reaction can be quantified by measuring the diameter of the wheal and associated erythema (Table 8-1).[3]
- Wheal size was found to be more specific than erythema size and to correlate better to clinical symptoms.
- The results should be measured at the peak of the reaction.[1]
  - ○ The peak time for histamine reaction is 8–10 minutes.
  - ○ The peak time for mast cell activators such as opiates is 10–15 minutes.
  - ○ The peak time for most allergen is 15–20 minutes.
- **Positive reactions are any wheals that measure >3 mm in diameter more than the negative control.**

Contraindications
- Skin tests should not be performed in patients who have had a **recent severe allergic reaction** (i.e., anaphylaxis) because test results are unreliable in these instances. Skin testing is usually postponed for 4–6 weeks after the acute event.

TABLE 8-1	GRADING SYSTEM FOR SKIN TESTING	
Prick test	**Intradermal test**	**Patch test**
1+: erythema <21 mm	1+: 3 to 4 mm wheal with erythema	0: (negative): no detectable change in appearance of skin
2+: erythema >20 mm	2+: 4 to 8 mm wheal without pseudopods	1+: erythema with edema covering at least ½ of test area
3+: wheal >3 mm	3+: wheal >8 mm without pseudopods	2+: erythema and edema plus papules
4+: wheal with pseudopods	4+: wheal with pseudopods	3+: vesicles and bullae plus erythema, edema, and papules

- Tests should not be performed on patients who have **severe eczema or dermatographism** because of difficulty in interpreting the results.[1]
- **Intradermal testing is never performed for food allergy.**[1,4]
- Skin testing should be performed with extreme caution in patients with a history of severe hypersensitivity reactions (i.e., to venom, foods, drugs) and usually not while patients are on β-adrenergic blocking agents.[1,5]

Interfering Medications

- Several medications can interfere with skin test results **usually due to antihistaminic effects.**
- The mean and maximum number of days of skin testing suppression differs for each medication based on its pharmacologic properties.
- While many medications can be stopped without major adverse effects, stopping other medications such as tricyclic antidepressants and atypical antipsychotics agents can lead to serious health consequences relating to the condition that is being treated.
- Table 8-2 includes a list of classes of medications and how long they should be discontinued before testing.[1]

Less Common Forms of Skin Testing

- **Scratch skin test:**
  - The scratch skin test is performed by making abrasions on the skin and then applying the allergen extract to the site, allowing it to diffuse through the skin.
  - Because of its **poor standardization and reproducibility,** this method has fallen out of favor and is rarely used.
- **Prausnitz–Kustner test:**
  - The Prausnitz–Kustner test is a passive transfer test and is of **historical interest only.**

TABLE 8-2	DRUGS THAT INTERFERE WITH ALLERGY SKIN TESTING	
Medication class	**Duration of skin test suppression**	**Comments**
Antihistamines (first or second generation)	2–3 days	Exceptions include cetirizine, hydroxyzine, and loratadine, which can persist for 5–7 days
Tricyclic antidepressants	7–10 days	
H_2 antihistamines	<1 day	
Cysteinyl leukotriene antagonists	No suppression	
Oral corticosteroids ≤30 mg prednisone <1 week	No suppression	
>20 mg prednisone >1 week	Possible suppression	
Topical corticosteroids (high potency)	3 weeks to the area of application	

Adapted from: Bernstein IL, Li JT, Bernstein DI, et al. Allergy diagnostic testing: an updated practice parameter. *Ann Allergy Asthma Immunol* 2008;100:S1–S48.

○ This test was the first method by which specific allergic sensitivities were determined before the knowledge of IgE.

○ The serum of a patient with a specific allergy (e.g., to eggs) would be taken and placed on the marked location on the skin of another, nonallergic person.

○ That same spot would be challenged later with the allergen (e.g., the egg protein) and a wheal-and-flare reaction would be observed.

○ Given the hazards of transmitting blood-borne disease from serum, this test is no longer used.

• **Set point titration:**

○ Set point titration is a method developed by Rinkel in which serial dilutions of extract are tested using the intradermal method.

○ Dilutions of allergenic extract increasing in fivefold concentrations are placed and observed for a wheal reaction.

○ A set point is defined as the testing dose that initiates an incremental 2 mm increase in the wheal with the fivefold increase in concentration.

○ There is controversy over the scientific validity of this testing method.

In Vitro Testing of IgE

Total Serum IgE

• The test measures total circulating IgE and not the amount of IgE responsible for clinical symptoms.[2]

• Total serum IgE can be helpful in identifying persons with high likelihood of atopy but **should not be used as a diagnostic or screening test on its own.**

• Difficulty of applying total IgE levels is partly due to their variance with age, especially in the pediatric population, and the considerable overlap between normal and atopic individuals.

• Thus, **mildly elevated levels of IgE are not generally helpful.**

• Usually, levels that are >1,800 IU/mL indicate a likely diagnosis of atopy, whereas levels <20 IU/mL make diagnosis of atopy unlikely.

• Total serum IgE may be elevated in conditions in which the role of IgE is well understood such as follows:

○ Asthma
○ Allergic rhinitis
○ Eczema
○ Anaphylaxis from drug, food, or venom
○ Bronchopulmonary aspergillosis

• Other conditions with increased total IgE of unknown significance include:

○ Tobacco use
○ Alcoholism
○ Parasitic infection
○ HIV
○ IgE multiple myeloma
○ Wiskott–Aldrich syndrome
○ Churg–Strauss vasculitis
○ Hyper-IgE syndrome (Job's syndrome)
○ Pemphigoid
○ Hodgkin's disease
○ Omenn's syndrome
○ Severe burns

TABLE 8-3	COMPARISON OF SKIN AND *IN VITRO* ALLERGY TESTING
Advantages of skin tests	**Advantages of *in vitro* tests**
Most sensitive in detection of antigen-specific IgE	No risk of anaphylaxis
Results available in minutes	Not affected by medications
Greater selection of allergens	Can be used on patient's with skin conditions that would preclude skin testing
Cheaper than *in vitro* tests	Convenient for patients afraid of needles
Minimal equipment needed	Perceived by patients as more scientific

In Vitro Methods of Detecting Antigen-specific IgE

- Antigen-specific IgE can also be detected using laboratory techniques.[2]
- Advantages and disadvantages of *in vivo* (i.e., skin testing, see above) and *in vitro* allergy testing can be found in Table 8-3.[1,2]
- All *in vitro* tests of antigen-specific IgE use the principle of immunoadsorption.
  ○ First, the antigen in question is bound to a solid phase (e.g., a paper disk, cellulose sponge, or plastic microtiter well plate).
  ○ A patient's serum is incubated with the solid phase.
  ○ After washing, a labeled anti-human IgE is incubated with the solid phase.
  ○ After another washing, the amount of labeled anti-IgE is measured and reported either in absolute IgE units or as a class score.
  ○ A class score of 0 is negative, scores in the range 0–1 are considered indeterminate, and any score >2 is considered positive and should be correlated with clinical history.
- Older methods used radiolabeled reagents to quantify absorbed antigen-specific IgE. This method is called radioallergosorbent test (RAST), a term that is still used to refer to any method of *in vitro* quantitation of antigen-specific IgE.
- Radiologic methods for quantitation of antigen-specific IgE have been largely replaced by fluorescence-based methods.

Diagnostic Testing for Allergic Contact Dermatitis: Patch Testing

- The patch skin test is the most useful tool in identifying the cause of allergic contact dermatitis.[2]
- Unlike epicutaneous and intradermal skin testing, patch testing is **a measure of a delayed hypersensitivity reaction or a cell-mediated hypersensitivity reaction.**[1,2]
- The test artificially attempts to reproduce the patient's clinical symptoms and helps determine provocative antigens.[2]
- It has limitations in that **the sensitivity and specificity are only 70%,** even when performed by the most experienced clinicians.
- While antihistamines are not contraindicated, **topical corticosteroids should not be applied to the patch test site** for several days before testing. High dose oral corticosteroids (>20 mg/day of prednisone) may also lead to false-negative results.
- **Oral corticosteroids should ideally be discontinued for 1 week before testing,** but sensitivity remains adequate even when chronic oral steroids are used at a dose of ≤15 mg prednisone per day.

Methods
- It is important to determine that the area of skin to be tested is **without irritation or inflammation.**[1,2]
- Small amounts of diluted testing materials are placed on small aluminum disks and are placed on the patient's back under nonocclusive dressing with hypoallergenic tape. Each test material's concentration should be sufficiently dilute to minimize the chance of an irritant reaction. Standard testing kits are also available commercially.
- **Two days after placing patch tests, the patient should return for removal of the disks and grading of the test areas.**
- The patient should not bathe, shower, or participate in strenuous activities until the test site is graded.
- **The patient should return for a late reading 4–5 days after original application.** The late reading will increase sensitivity because some reactions may not be evident at the first reading.

Precautions
- The application of the patch test may itself sensitize the patient or cause a flare-up in an already-sensitized patient.[1]
- Patients should be instructed to remove any patch that is causing severe irritation. Repeated patch testing should be avoided.
- Standardized concentrations of test material should be used to avoid an inflammatory reaction, and thus a false-positive result.

Allergen Panels
- Only 28 commercially prepared allergens are FDA-approved in the United States.
- There are several patch test kits containing these allergens; one is described in Table 8-4.[6] Note that one component is a negative control.
- While the 28 commercially prepared allergens are convenient to use, they only detect 25–30% of all cases of allergic contact dermatitis. As a result, the North American Contact Dermatitis Group commonly tests for 65 allergens, but most of these are not FDA-approved and therefore cannot be commercially purchased.[1]

Grading
- Each reagent is graded on a scale of 0–3 as presented in Table 8-1.[1]
- Grades 1+ and above are considered positive.
- False-positive test results may be due to the following:
  - Skin may be hypersensitive to one of the antigens, and, therefore, the entire back can become inflamed.
  - Irritation due to factors other than antigen (i.e., the tape used).
- False-negative test results may be due to the following:
  - Concentration of antigen was too low.
  - Technical errors in applying the antigen patches.
  - Late reading at 3–7 days not performed.

Clinical Application of Test Results
- It is important to remember that **a positive patch skin test result does not mean diagnosis of causative agent for contact dermatitis.**[1]
- The antigen could be a secondary aggravating factor.
- Positive test results should be correlated with clinical history, and, when possible, the patient should avoid the antigens that caused a positive reaction.

TABLE 8-4   T.R.U.E. TEST PANEL OF ALLERGENS[a]

Allergen	Environmental occurrences
Nickel sulfate	Jewelry, metal
Wool alcohols (lanolin)	Cosmetics, soaps, topical medications
Neomycin sulfate	Topical antibiotics
Potassium dichromate	Cement, cutting oils
Caine mix	Topical anesthetics
Fragrance mix	Toiletries, scented household products
Colophony	Cosmetics, adhesives
Paraben mix	Preservative in topical formulations and foods
Negative control	—
Balsam of Peru	Foods, cosmetics
Ethylenediamine dihydrochloride	Topical medicines, industrial solvents
Cobalt dichloride	Metal-plated objects, paints
p-tert-Butylphenol formaldehyde resin	Waterproof glues, bonded leather
Epoxy resin	Two-part adhesives, paints
Carba mix	Rubber products, glues for leather, vinyl
Black rubber mix	All black rubber products, some hair dyes
Cl+ Me– isothiazolinone	Cosmetics, topical medicines
Quaternium-15	Preservative in cosmetics, household cleaners
Mercaptobenzothiazole	Rubber products, adhesives
p-Phenylenediamine	Hair dyes, dyed textiles
Formaldehyde	Fabric finishes, plastics, synthetic resins
Mercapto mix	Rubber products, glues for leather/plastics
Thimerosal	Preservative in contact lens solutions and injectable drugs
Thiuram mix	Rubber products, adhesives
Diazolidinyl urea	Cosmetics, cleaning agents, liquid soaps, pet shampoos
Imidazolidinyl urea	Cosmetics, cleaning agents, liquid soaps, moisturizers
Budesonide	Topical, inhaled, and rectal anti-inflammatory agent
Tixocortol-21-pivalate	Anti-inflammatory agents such as nasal spray, lozenges, and rectal suspensions
Quinoline mix	Topical antibiotic and antifungal preparations; animal food

Adapted from: www.truetest.com/panelallergens.aspx.
[a]See the website for specific information including concentrations of each allergen and cross-reactivity.

REFERENCES

1. Bernstein IL, Li JT, Bernstein DI, et al. Allergy diagnostic testing: an updated practice parameter. *Ann Allergy Asthma Immunol* 2008;100:S1–S48.
2. Demoly P, Bousquet J, Ramano A. *Middleton's Allergy Principles and Practice,* Vol. 2, 7th ed. Mosby, MO: Maryland Heights, 2009; Chapter 71.
3. Nelson H. Clinical application of immediate skin testing. In: Spector SL, ed. *Provocative Challenge Procedures: Background and Methodology.* Armonk, NY: Futura, 1989:647.
4. Bock SA, Lee WY, Remigio L, et al. Appraisal of skin tests with food extracts for diagnosis of food hypersensitivity. *Clin Allergy* 1978;8:559–564.
5. Lieberman P, Nicklas RA, Oppenheimer J, et al. The diagnosis and management of anaphylaxis practice parameter: 2010 update. *J Allergy Clin Immunol* 2010;126:477–480.
6. T.R.U.E. Test Allergen Patch. www.truetest.com/panelallergens.aspx. Accessed 9/30/11.

Urticaria and Angioedema

9

James A. Tarbox

GENERAL PRINCIPLES

- Urticaria and angioedema are commonly seen conditions of heterogeneous origin.
- A detailed history is the most important factor in determining etiology.
- Hereditary angioedema (HAE) is quite rare with initial screening showing a low C4 level.
- Nonsedating H1 antihistamines are the main stay of therapy.
- While acute urticaria/angioedema is self-limiting, chronic urticaria/angioedema may last years without treatment.

Definition

- **Urticaria** is defined as raised, round areas of edema (wheal) surrounded by reflex erythema (flare) that involves only the superficial dermis of the skin.
- The lesions are usually pruritic and may develop rapidly. Any single lesion **does not ordinarily last >24 hours.**
- **Angioedema** extends into the deep dermis or subcutaneous tissue and often affects areas of loose connective tissue, such as the face.
  ○ Angioedema may be uncomfortable or painful rather than pruritic, especially when the viscera are involved, and can last for several days.
  ○ Angioedema involving a patient's larynx can threaten the airway and lead to asphyxiation.

Classification

- Although lesions of urticaria/angioedema are histologically the same regardless of the cause, differences in etiology and therapy warrant the classification into acute and chronic syndromes.
- The syndrome is defined as **acute** if the lesions are of **<6 weeks** duration.[1]
- **Chronic** urticaria/angioedema has lesions that have lasted **>6 weeks.** The syndrome lasts an average of 3–5 years, with 20% of patients still symptomatic at 20 years.[2]
  ○ In recent years, it has been demonstrated that many patients with chronic urticaria exhibit autoantibodies directed against the high-affinity immunoglobulin E (IgE) receptor.
  ○ In addition to autoimmune urticaria, several physical urticaria syndromes are important to define, because once diagnosed, no further workup is usually necessary.

Epidemiology

- 15–24% of the US population will experience urticaria or angioedema at some time in their life.[1]
- Urticaria is often a symptom of another allergic disorder such as anaphylaxis or food allergy.

- When presenting as part of another allergic syndrome, urticaria is generally considered a secondary diagnosis.
- Most cases of isolated urticaria are mild and self-limited.
- Chronic idiopathic urticaria (CIU) is common, affecting about 3% of the population with an economic and social burden comparable to that seen with severe coronary artery disease.[3]
- Angioedema occurs in approximately 50% of the cases of chronic urticaria, while about 10% of the individuals experience angioedema without hives.[4]
- Chronic urticaria is more common in adults and women.

Etiology

Acute Urticaria and Angioedema
- Many infections, especially viral infections, may be accompanied by self-limited urticaria.
- Allergic reactions to medications are a common cause of acute urticaria.
  - **Penicillin and cephalosporin** class IgE-mediated reactions.
  - **Sulfonamides and platinum-based chemotherapy** (i.e., oxaliplatin).
  - **Nonsteroidal antiinflammatory drugs (NSAIDS) and angiotensin-converting enzyme (ACE) inhibitors** are the most common cause of non–IgE-mediated reactions.
- Food allergy is often associated with urticaria. Peanuts, tree nuts, and shellfish are the most common causes in adults.
- Insect stings.

Chronic Urticaria and Angioedema
- Causes of chronic urticaria and angioedema include[5]:
  - CIU
  - **Autoimmune urticaria:** Autoimmunity to IgE receptor or IgE:
    - IgG against IgE or the IgE receptor is reported between 30 and 40%.[6]
    - Association with antithyroid antibodies
  - Physical urticarias and angioedema
  - Drugs
  - Food and food additives
  - Aeroallergens and contactants
  - Infections
  - Systemic immune-mediated diseases and vasculitis
- If physically induced urticarias are excluded, the incidence of identifying an external allergen responsible for chronic urticaria is <5%.[6]

Acquired Angioedema
- B-cell lymphoproliferative disease
- T-cell lymphoma
- Multiple myeloma
- Myelofibrosis

Pathophysiology

Acute Urticaria and Angioedema
- Acute urticaria caused by a known exposure (e.g., drugs, food, stings) is caused by **cross-linking of antigen-specific IgE** on the surface of mast cells leading to **inflammatory mediator release.**

- **Histamine** is the principal mediator of urticaria and angioedema; however, many other mediators, such as prostaglandin D_2, leukotrienes C and D, platelet-activating factor, and components of the complement and coagulation cascades, can be involved. This complexity explains why antihistamines sometimes may not be completely effective.
- Although the **mast cell is the major effector in all forms of urticaria and angioedema,** other cells, such as the basophil, are also involved.
- Urticaria and angioedema may also result from direct mast cell stimulation (as in reactions to radiocontrast media or opiate drugs), as well as components of the complement and arachidonic acid pathways.

Autoimmune Chronic Urticaria
- Studies have shown a subset of patients with CIU have autoantibodies directed against the high-affinity IgE receptor, IgE, thyroglobulin, or thyroperoxidase.
- In the majority of patients with CIU no etiology is identified.

Hereditary Angioedema
- HAE is caused by **lack or dysfunction of C1 esterase inhibitor (C1-INH)** and is characterized by periodic attacks of angioedema that are often, but not always, triggered by trauma (i.e., dental surgery).
- The majority of patients possess an **autosomal dominant** mutation in the gene encoding C1-INH.
- Lack of C1-INH results in **accumulation of bradykinin**, which is the main mediator responsible symptoms in HAE.

Acquired C1q Angioedema
Development of autoantibodies to C1q results in a clinical syndrome very similar to HAE, but distinguishable by the lack of C1q.

Urticarial Vasculitis
Immune complex deposition within cutaneous blood vessels can result in recruitment of complement and cause a leukocytoclastic vasculitis manifesting as urticaria.

Associated Conditions
- Urticarial vasculitis is associated with numerous conditions, including collagen vascular disease, chronic hepatitis, Lyme disease, myelomas, and cryoglobulinemias, as well as others.
- Anaphylaxis
- Thyroid autoimmunity

DIAGNOSIS

Clinical Presentation
- Urticaria is characterized by the sudden appearance of wheals and/or angioedema.[7]
- A wheal consists of three typical features:
  - Central swelling of variable size, almost invariably surrounded by a reflex erythema
  - Associated itching or, sometimes, burning sensation
  - Fleeting nature, with the skin returning to its normal appearance, usually within 1–24 hours

- Angioedema is characterized by:
  - Sudden, pronounced swelling of the lower dermis and subcutis.
  - Sometimes pain rather than itching.
  - Frequent involvement below mucous membranes.
  - Resolution that is slower than for wheals and can take up to 72 hours.

Acute Urticaria and Angioedema

- **Drug reactions:** All current and recent prescription and over-the-counter medications and herbal supplements must be scrutinized.
- **The most common drugs causing hives are antibiotics and opiate analgesics.**
- **ACE inhibitors, nonselective beta-blockers, aspirin, and NSAIDs** may cause or exacerbate urticaria and/or angioedema.
- There are sporadic cases of specific NSAIDs causing urticaria, but, in general, all NSAIDs cross-react.
- **Food ingestions:** Fish, milk, eggs, wheat, soy, nuts, and peanuts are the most common foods causing urticaria, although a person may develop an allergy to potentially any food (see Chap. 16).
- **Physical stimuli:** Related to lesions (see the section on Physical Urticaria Syndromes).
- **Evidence of infection:** Viral hepatitis, mononucleosis, fungal infections, helminthes (usually accompanied by high eosinophilia) have all been associated with urticaria. There may be an association between *Helicobacter pylori* infection and urticaria, but this relationship remains controversial.
- **Aeroallergen:** Rarely, patients with seasonal allergies experience urticaria/angioedema during episodes of high exposure.
- **Recent sting or insect bite:** See Chapter 15.
- **Food additives:** Rare causes of urticaria/angioedema, but reactions to some food additives and dyes have been reported (see Chapter 16).
- **Family history of similar lesions:** Consider HAE or a familial urticarial syndrome.
- **Review of systems** for collagen vascular disease, hepatic disease, autoimmune thyroiditis, lymphoproliferative disorders, and malignancy. The latter two are associated with acquired C1 inhibitor deficiency.

Chronic Urticaria

- While it is rare to identify a causative antigen in chronic urticaria, a complete history is essential to rule out environmental exposures.
- Chronic urticaria can occasionally be a symptom of an underlying systemic disease such as autoimmunity or infection, so evaluating the patient's complete medical history is important.
- Any single urticarial lesion usually lasts <24 hours.
- If lesions last longer, consider urticarial vasculitis, delayed pressure urticaria or an alternative diagnosis.

Hereditary Angioedema

- Characteristic presentation is recurrent swelling beginning in adolescence.
- Can involve nearly any part of the body, including the larynx, and usually lasts several days.
- When involving the viscera, HAE can present similarly to small bowel obstruction.
- **Episodes are virtually never associated with urticaria.**
- There will often, but not always, be a family history angioedema.

Physical Urticarias

- **Cold urticaria**
  - Seen on **cold, exposed areas of skin.**
  - Fatalities have been reported from hypotension occurring while swimming.
  - Secondary acquired cold urticaria is related to cryoglobulins resulting from systemic disease (hepatitis B or C) or lymphoreticular malignancy.
- **Cholinergic (heat) urticaria**
  - Related to **elevated core temperature** from exercise, a hot shower, or emotional stress.
  - Lesions are typically tiny and diffuse.
  - Occurs in approximately 15% of the population.
  - Severe forms may progress to angioedema and syncope although lesions usually resolve if the patient "cools off."
- **Dermographism**
  - Literally "skin writing" is another common form of physical urticaria.
  - Affects approximately 4% of the population.
  - Can be elicited on examining by briskly stroking skin with tongue blade or fingernail.
  - May confound ability to read allergen skin tests.
  - Lesions are transitory and respond to suppression with antihistamines.
- **Delayed pressure urticaria/angioedema**
  - Unlike other physical urticaria, lesions appear **4–6 hours after the stimulus of pressure.**
  - Mediators are thought to be similar to late-phase reactants rather than histamine.
  - Poorly responsive to antihistamines; systemic steroids may be needed to control severely afflicted patients.
- **Vibratory urticaria**
  - Rare disorder usually occurs in patients exposed to persistent vibrations, such as drills or pneumatic hammers.
- **Solar urticaria**
  - The history usually establishes the diagnosis of this very rare disorder.
  - Different categories depending on wavelength of light-producing symptoms.
- **Aquagenic urticaria**
  - This form of physical urticaria is exceedingly rare.
  - Patients react to a wet compress regardless of its temperature.

Other Urticarias

- **Exercise-induced urticaria**
  - Different from cholinergic urticaria in that it is **not related to core body temperature.**
  - **Lesions are typically urticarial and progress to anaphylaxis.**
  - In some patients, the ingestion of a specific food before exercise is necessary (e.g., celery) to trigger the reaction, although eating before exercise in general will worsen symptoms in most patients.
- **Urticarial vasculitis**
  - Examination usually reveals lesions in dependent areas.
  - Other signs of vasculitis, such as petechiae and palpable purpura, are often evident.
  - Lesions tend to **last >24 hours** and be more painful than pruritic.

Differential Diagnosis

- **Erythema multiforme minor:** Lesions persist rather than wax/wane. Lesions are usually preceded by a prodrome of constitutional symptoms.
- **Bullous pemphigoid and dermatitis herpetiformis:** Initial presentation may be similar but the formation of bullae rules out urticaria.
- **Mastocytosis:** Characteristic lesions of urticaria pigmentosa, mastocytoma, and telangiectasia eruptive macularis perstans (TEMP) (see Chap. 19).
- **Muckle–Wells syndrome:** A rare autosomal dominant autoinflammatory syndrome characterized by sensorineural deafness, recurrent urticaria, fevers, arthritis, and amyloidosis.
- **Schnitzler's syndrome:** Usually presents with chronic nonpruritic urticaria, recurrent fever, and arthritis and is accompanied by a monoclonal gammopathy.
- **Gleich's syndrome** (episodic angioedema with eosinophilia): Characterized by episodic angioedema with findings of an IgM gammopathy and eosinophilia on laboratory testing.

Diagnostic Testing

- **Acute urticaria**
  - Cause of episode, if identifiable, is usually established by history.
  - When caused by a food or medication, the presence of an antigen-specific IgE, demonstrated by either *in vivo* or *in vitro* testing (see Chap. 8), confirms diagnosis.
  - Food diaries may be helpful in direct specific IgE tests.
- **Autoimmune chronic urticaria**
  - A subset of patients with chronic idiopathic urticaria have autoantibodies directed against the high-affinity IgE receptor, thyroglobulin, or thyroperoxidase. The **CU Index (anti-FcεRI antibody)** can be used to demonstrate the presence of autoantibodies that potentially could cause chronic urticaria.
  - In some patients, autologous skin testing (using the patient's serum) is positive. However, this is not diagnostic, as these autoantibodies can be seen in other disease states and in some normal patients.
  - Other laboratories often sent to rule out systemic illnesses causing disease include: antithyroid antibodies against thyroperoxidase and thyroglobulin, thyroid-stimulating hormone (TSH), complete blood count (CBC), urinalysis, erythrocyte sedimentation rate (ESR), liver function tests, and antinuclear antibodies (ANA).
- **Urticarial vasculitis: A punch biopsy is necessary to make the diagnosis** and will show leukocytoclastic vasculitis.
- **HAE:** Diagnosis is made by an initial screening C4 level that is always low and can drop to undetectable levels during an attack.
  - If the C4 level is low, obtain a C1 inhibitor level. In approximately 15–20% of patients, the level is normal, but the protein is not functional, and a functional assay must be performed.
- **Acquired angioedema:** A low C1q level combined with low C1 inhibitor and C4 levels warrants an investigation for an occult malignancy, because this disorder is associated with lymphoproliferative disorders. It is also rarely associated with connective tissue disease.
- **Cold urticaria:** Test with an ice cube on forearm for 3 minutes; the lesions seen on re-warming.

- **Cholinergic (heat) urticaria:** Test by running vigorously in place for 10 minutes or submersion in warm water.
- **Dermographism:** Briskly stroke skin with tongue blade or fingernail. Note linear lesions from excoriation on exam.
- **Pressure urticaria/angioedema:** Test with 15 lb weight in a sling over forearm.
- **Vibratory urticaria:** Test by holding patient's forearm on a lab vortex for 4 minutes or using a tuning fork.

TREATMENT

Urticaria and Angioedema

- Choice of treatment depends on the etiology of the lesions. It may involve avoidance (as in NSAIDs or opiates), treatment of an underlying condition (such as thyroid replacement for autoimmune thyroiditis), or medications.
- Treatment for physical urticarias includes avoiding triggers of the underlying disorder.
- For both chronic and acute forms of urticaria angioedema, **avoidance of possible triggers, when identified, is a key to treatment.**
- Second-generation (nonsedating) H1 blocking antihistamines are first-line medication in treatment of symptomatic urticaria and angioedema (Appendix A, Table A-1).
- Self-injectable epinephrine should be prescribed for any patient with airway compromising angioedema.
- First-generation (sedating) H1 blocking antihistamines (Appendix A, Table A-1) are often helpful, particularly if symptoms are worse at night.
- **Doxepin,** a tricyclic antidepressant with strong antihistaminic effects, is often used for nighttime symptoms.
  - The typical starting dose is 10 mg at bedtime.
  - Doxepin can be very sedating; caution regarding daytime somnolence and slowed reaction times is warranted.
- **Second-line medications** include the following:
  - **H2 blocking antihistamines**
    - Ranitidine: 150 mg twice daily
    - Cimetidine: 400 mg twice daily (use with caution because of medication interactions)
  - **Leukotriene modifiers** (e.g., montelukast)
- Many patients with urticaria require **more than one class of medication** to control their symptoms (e.g., H1 antihistamine in combination with H2 antihistamines).
- A short burst of **prednisone** can often eradicate symptoms but has numerous, well-documented side effects. Therefore, steroids should be used in severe cases or in cases refractory to antihistamines.
  - The dose and course should be high enough and long enough to control symptoms.
  - Tapering steroids is not necessary to prevent adrenal suppression for short courses but can be helpful to determine if symptoms have remitted and to achieve the lowest effective dose.
  - Typical doses are 40–60 mg/day for severe exacerbations.
  - Patients should be adequately counseled regarding side effects associated with steroids.

- **Cyclosporine,** a calcineurin inhibitor often used to prevent transplant rejection, has been shown to have efficacy in treating both chronic idiopathic and autoimmune urticaria.[8]
  - Cyclosporine should only be used by experienced clinicians.
  - CBC, complete metabolic profile (CMP), urinalysis, and cyclosporine trough levels must be routinely monitored.
- Dapsone, plaquenil, and other immunosuppressive agents have been used with varying success for chronic urticaria refractory to other treatments.

Hereditary Angioedema

- The approach to treatment of HAE is distinct from allergic angioedema.
- Acute management of HAE is directed at stabilizing the patient and reducing the extent of swelling.
  - Angioedema involving the airway is a major mortality risk for patients with HAE.
  - Elective **intubation must be considered** if swelling is involving the airway.
  - **Fluid resuscitation** may be necessary due to third spacing.
  - Medications for acute HAE attacks include:
    - **Human C1-INH** (Berinert), which is a plasma-derived concentrate of C1-INH, is an FDA-approved for treatment of acute abdominal or facial attacks of HAE.[9]
    - **Ecallantide** (Kalbitor) is a reversible inhibitor of plasma kallikrein that has been shown to be effective for acute attacks of swelling in HAE.[10]
    - Debate exists regarding the use of fresh frozen plasma during an acute attack, as this has been seen to worsen symptoms in a few patients.
    - Epinephrine has often been used for attacks, but there are no studies to support its efficacy.
    - **The use of antihistamines and corticosteroids are of little value.**
- Chronic treatment of HAE focuses on preventing angioedema episodes.
  - **Synthetic androgenic steroids** (danazol or stanozolol) increase the synthesis of C1 inhibitor and can prevent angioedema episodes. Despite having attenuated virilizing side effects, these agents can have side effects and should not be used in pregnant woman.
  - **Fibrinolytic agents** (such as ε-aminocaproic acid) have also been shown to ameliorate symptoms. Unfortunately, this therapy also carries the risk of numerous side effects.
  - **Human C1-INH** (Cinryze) is also approved to help prevent angioedema attacks in teenagers and adults with HAE.[11]

OUTCOME/PROGNOSIS

- The prognosis of urticaria depends on its etiology.
- Patients with acute urticaria from an identifiable exposure have an excellent prognosis with strict avoidance of the provoking antigen.
- In cases of acute urticaria without identifiable cause, most patients have resolution of symptoms within 6 weeks of onset. A small subset of these patients will go on to develop CIU.
- Most patients with CIU have eventual resolution of their symptoms—usually over the course of years. Cyclosporine may speed the resolution of chronic urticaria.

- Patient with unexplained or difficult to manage acute urticaria/angioedema and chronic urticaria/angioedema should be referred to allergy and immunology for further management.

REFERENCES

1. Joint Task Force on Practice Parameters. The diagnosis and management of urticaria: a practice parameter part I: acute urticaria/angioedema part II: chronic urticaria/angioedema. joint task force on practice parameters. *Ann Allergy Asthma Immunol* 2000;85:521–544.
2. Najib U, Sheikh J. An update on acute and chronic urticaria for the primary care provider. *Postgrad Med* 2009;121:141–151.
3. O'Donnell BF, Lawlor F, Simpson J, et al. The impact of chronic urticaria on the quality of life. *Br J Dermatol* 1997;136:197–201.
4. Fox RW. Chronic urticaria and/or angioedema. *Clin Rev Allergy Immunol* 2002;23:143–145.
5. Kulczycki A. Urticaria and angioedema. In: Elizabeth GN, David AF, eds. *ACP Medicine.* 4th ed. Hamilton, OH: BC Decker Inc., 2010.
6. Kikuchi Y, Kaplan AP. Mechanisms of autoimmune activation of basophils in chronic urticaria. *J Allergy Clin Immunol* 2001;107:1056–1062.
7. Zuberbier T, Asero R, Bindslev-Jensen C, et al. EAACI/GA(2)LEN/EDF/WAO guideline: definition, classification and diagnosis of urticaria. *Allergy* 2009;64:1417–1426.
8. Kessel A, Toubi E. Cyclosporine-A in severe chronic urticaria: the option for long-term therapy. *Allergy* 2010;65:1478–1482.
9. Craig TJ, Lew RJ, Wasserman RL, et al. Efficacy of human C1 esterase inhibitor concentrate compared with placebo in acute hereditary angioedema attacks. *J Allergy Clin Immunol* 2009;124:801–808.
10. Sheffer AL, Campion M, Lew RJ, et al. Ecallantide (DX-88) for acute hereditary angioedema attacks: integrated analysis of 2 double-blind, phase 3 studies. *J Allergy Clin Immunol* 2011;128:153–159.
11. Zuraw BL, Busse PJ, White M, et al. Nanofiltered C1 inhibitor concentrate for treatment of hereditary angioedema. *N Engl J Med* 2010;363:513–522.

Atopic Dermatitis

Amanda Trott

GENERAL PRINCIPLES

- Atopic dermatitis (AD) is the most common chronic skin disease of young children, affecting 17% of US schoolchildren and a significant number of adults.[1]
- Both skin and immune system genes play a key role, and immune defects may result in colonization and infection by microbial organisms.

Definition

- AD is a **chronically relapsing skin disease** that is usually associated with respiratory allergy. It involves the local infiltration of T_H2 cells (see Chapter 2), which is the same type of inflammatory response seen in asthma and allergic rhinitis.
- AD can result in significant morbidity, and the cause remains unknown, although it is understood to involve a complex interrelationship of genetic, environmental, immunologic, and epidermal mechanisms.

Epidemiology

- AD affects a **higher proportion of children than adults.**
  - 90% of patients with AD develop symptoms before the age of 5.[1]
  - The majority of children affected by AD appear to outgrow this inflammatory skin disease.[2]
- Multiple studies suggest that the population percentage affected by AD is on the rise.
  - A Japanese study found a twofold increase in AD prevalence in 9- to 12-year olds when compared to similarly aged children examined 20 years earlier.[3]
  - This increased frequency is not unique to AD and is paralleled by increase in the prevalence of other atopic diseases, such as allergic rhinitis and asthma.
  - Possible reasons for this include greater exposure to pollutants and indoor allergens, decreased breast-feeding, and increased awareness of AD.

Etiology

- **Genetics** of AD are complex, and research is evolving our understanding of AD.
  - Compromise of the epidermal barrier, which can occur through various mechanisms, is thought to lead to increased water loss and facilitates entry of allergens and microbes.
  - Mutations in filaggrin, a protein involved in keratinization of the skin and in barrier function maintenance, have been demonstrated to be a major predisposing factor for a significant subset of patients with AD.[4]
  - Mutations in protease inhibitors (SPINK5) are also linked to AD. These mutations are thought to lead an imbalance of proteolytic activity that results in barrier compromise.[5]

- Most patients with AD have an **atopic predisposition** and develop an immuno-globulin E (IgE) response to common environmental allergens.
  - Elevated IgE and positive reaction to allergens upon skin testing are seen in up to 85% of patients with AD.[1]
    - Atopy results in overproduction of T_H2-type cytokines, resulting in eosino-philia.
    - Allergic inflammation causes intrinsic hyperreactivity of inflammatory cells resulting in lower threshold for irritation.
  - Exposure to food allergens and aeroallergens can cause exacerbations in some patients with AD.
  - AD predominantly of the head and neck is often associated with positive testing to certain fungal organisms and may improve with antifungal therapy.
- The majority of patients with severe AD have IgE against human proteins (autoantigens).

Pathophysiology

- The immunologic basis for AD is supported by evidence showing patients with primary immunodeficiency disorders whose eczema either corrects after bone marrow transplant, or who develop AD after successful engraftment from an atopic donor.
- Additionally, there are immunoregulatory differences seen in patients with AD.[6]
  - T cells produce more interleukin (IL)-4 and express higher levels of IL-4 receptor.
  - Increased numbers of T_H2 cells secreting IL-4, IL-5, and IL-13 after allergen exposure, resulting in:
    - Inhibition of interferon (IFN)-γ production by mononuclear cells.
    - Increased IgE synthesis by B cells.
    - Migration, differentiation, and proliferation of eosinophils.
- Inflammation in AD is characterized by:
  - Monocytes secreting more prostaglandin E2 and IL-10, both of which inhibit IFN-γ (a T_H1 cytokine).
  - Langerhans cells and macrophages infiltrating into the skin lesion with surface-bound IgE. These cells do not typically have surface IgE in patients without AD.
  - Neutrophils are absent in skin biopsies of AD, which is a result of defective chemotactic activity. This partially explains the increased frequency of cutaneous infections.
  - Activated eosinophils are typically prominent in chronic AD lesions.
  - Keratinocytes secrete pro-inflammatory cytokines such as thymic stromal lymphopoietin (TSLP), while also producing reduced amounts of antimicrobial peptides.[7]
  - Reduced production of antimicrobial peptide and cytokines predisposes patients to greater infection and colonization with *Staphylococcus aureus,* viruses, and fungi.[8]
- IgE has multiple roles in AD:
  - Immediate response of pruritus and erythema after allergen exposure is a result of degranulation of mast cells bearing allergen-specific IgE.
  - Antigen presentation is potentiated by epidermal Langerhans cells expressing IgE on their surface.
- Chronic inflammation in AD is the result of multiple factors:
  - Repeated exposure to allergens leads to T_H2-type cell expansion.

- Monocytes in patients with AD have lower incidence of apoptosis, which results in increased production of factors promoting T_H2-type inflammatory response.
- Allergen-induced inflammation alters corticosteroid receptor binding affinity, which blunts the antiinflammatory effects of corticosteroids.
- Scratching injures keratinocytes, leading to their cytokine release and attraction of cells to the inflammatory site.

DIAGNOSIS

Clinical Presentation

History
- **Atopic diseases tend to cluster in individuals and in families,** so careful history taking regarding such diseases is very helpful.
  - Major risk factors for AD include either a family or personal history of atopic conditions, including AD, asthma, food allergy, and allergic rhinitis.
  - These four conditions are often referred to as the "allergic march of childhood."
  - AD and food allergy typically appear first and reach their highest prevalence within the first 2 years after birth.
- Careful history taking for **identification of environmental exposures** that worsen symptoms is an important part of the history.

Physical Examination
- Unaffected skin usually appears dry.
- **There are no pathognomonic skin lesions.**
- Acute AD is intensely pruritic and manifests with **erythematous papules with excoriations, vesicles, and serous exudate.**
- Chronic AD demonstrates thickened skin with **lichenification and fibrotic papules.**
- Distribution is usually a characteristic feature of AD.
  - In infants the face, scalp, and extensor surfaces of extremities are affected with sparing of the diaper area.
  - In children, involvement of the infragluteal area is common.
  - In older patients, involvement of the **flexural folds of extremities, hands, and feet** are common.

Diagnostic Criteria
- The diagnosis of AD is based on the presence of a constellation of clinical features.
- Major features:
  - Pruritus (presence critical for diagnosis).
  - Facial and extensor involvement in infants and children.
  - Flexural lichenification in adults.
  - Chronic or relapsing dermatitis.
  - Personal or family history of atopy.
- Minor features:
  - Xerosis.
  - Cutaneous infections.
  - Nonspecific dermatitis of the hands or feet.
  - Ichthyosis.
  - Palmar hyperlinearity.

- ○ Keratosis pilaris.
- ○ Pityriasis alba.
- ○ Nipple eczema.
- ○ Anterior subcapsular cataracts.
- ○ Elevated serum IgE levels.
- ○ Positive immediate-type allergy skin tests.

Differential Diagnosis

- Immunodeficiency should be considered, especially when AD presents in infancy:
  - ○ Immune dysregulation, polyendocrinopathy, enteropathy, and X-linked (IPEX) syndrome.
  - ○ Wiskott–Aldrich syndrome.
  - ○ Hyper-IgE syndrome.
  - ○ Severe combined immunodeficiency (SCID).
- Chronic dermatoses can often be differentiated from AD by history:
  - ○ Seborrheic dermatitis.
  - ○ Contact dermatitis.
  - ○ Nummular eczema.
  - ○ Lichen simplex chronicus.
- Infections:
  - ○ Scabies.
  - ○ HIV.
- Malignancy:
  - ○ Cutaneous T-cell lymphoma should be ruled out in an adult without history of childhood eczema.

Diagnostic Testing

Laboratories

- Laboratory tests are of limited value in diagnosis and management of AD. There are no **definitive diagnostic laboratories for AD.**
  - ○ Total IgE is frequently elevated in AD (but may be normal).
  - ○ Complete blood count (CBC) may show eosinophilia.
- Food-specific IgE concentrations do not identify the type or severity of the reaction and are therefore not very helpful in AD.
  - ○ *In vitro* measurement of antigen-specific IgE may occasionally be necessary if skin tests are not feasible or contraindicated (e.g., diffuse skin lesions or strong history of food-induced anaphylaxis).

Diagnostic Procedures

- Immediate hypersensitivity skin testing can be important in identifying environmental allergens contributing to comorbid conditions such as allergic rhinitis.
- In scenarios where a food antigen is suspected of contributing to AD, skin testing can be useful.
  - ○ **Negative testing with proper controls has a high predictive value for ruling out a suspected allergen** (i.e., excellent negative predictive value).
  - ○ In contrast, **positive tests have a poor correlation with clinical symptoms** in suspected food allergen–induced AD.
  - ○ Positive skin tests to foods suspected of contributing to AD should be confirmed with a **double-blind, placebo-controlled food challenge,** unless there is a history of anaphylaxis to the suspected food.

TREATMENT

Medications

First Line

- **Corticosteroids** work primarily as an antiinflammatory medication.
- They are effective for reducing inflammation and pruritus in both the acute and the chronic forms of AD.
- **The agent with the lowest effective potency should be used.**
- Although side effects of appropriately used low- to medium-potency topical corticosteroids are infrequent, problems such as thinning of the skin and hypopigmentation may occur, especially on the face and intertriginous areas.
- If a high-potency corticosteroid is indicated for a short time period, the patient must be provided with a lower-potency option for maintenance therapy to avoid flares.
- Once control is achieved with a daily corticosteroid regimen, **twice weekly application of the corticosteroid to the previously involved areas results in fewer relapses.**[9]
- Once daily treatment has shown to be effective with fluticasone propionate as well as mometasone furoate.
- Topical steroids are available in various bases, but **ointments have been shown to provide the best medication delivery while preventing evaporative losses.**
- Inadequate prescription size leads to suboptimally controlled AD.
- Topical steroids also decrease *S. aureus* colonization in patients with AD.[10]
- **Systemic corticosteroids should be avoided**, as they are often associated with significant flaring after discontinuation.

Second Line

- **Topical calcineurin inhibitors:**
  - These include tacrolimus ointment and pimecrolimus cream.
  - Although some patients complain of a transient burning sensation, these medications are not associated with skin atrophy and are therefore especially useful for treatment of the face and intertriginous regions.
  - Studies have shown that treatment with pimecrolimus cream upon early signs of AD results in a significantly decreased incidence of flares and need for topical corticosteroid rescue.[11]
- **Tar:**
  - Crude coal tar extracts have antiinflammatory properties that, when used with topical corticosteroids in chronic AD, may reduce the need for more potent corticosteroids.
  - Tar shampoos are often beneficial when the scalp is involved.
- **Oral cyclosporine A:** Placebo-controlled studies have demonstrated benefit of oral cyclosporine A in adults with severe AD.[12]
- **Azathioprine:**
  - Azathioprine is a systemic immunosuppressive agent that has been shown to be effective for severe recalcitrant AD.[12]
  - Its use is limited by a number of side effects and slow onset of action.
  - It is metabolized by thiopurine methyltransferase, so deficiency of this enzyme should be ruled out before initiation of treatment.

Antiinfective Therapy

- AD secondarily infected with *S. aureus* must be treated with 7–10 days of either semi-synthetic penicillins or first- or second-generation cephalosporins.

- If the area involved is localized, topical mupirocin applied three times daily for 7–10 days may be effective.
- Intranasal application of topical mupirocin twice daily for 5 days may reduce nasal carriage.
- Disseminated eczema herpeticum should be treated with systemic acyclovir.
- Superficial dermatophytosis can usually be treated with topical antifungal agents.

Antipruritic Agents
- Systemic antihistamines and anxiolytics are especially useful in the evening.
- Doxepin binds histamine receptors and can be given to adults before bed.
- Second-generation antihistamines have shown only modest clinical benefit in treating the pruritus associated with AD.
- Topical antihistamines and topical anesthetics should be avoided due to the risk of sensitization.

Other Nonpharmacologic Therapies

Trigger Avoidance
- **Irritants** are chemicals or other exposures that can nonspecifically worsen AD (**IgE-independent**).
  - Use cleansers with minimal defatting activity and a neutral pH rather than soaps.
  - Launder new clothing before wearing to reduce chemical content.
  - Use a liquid rather than a powder detergent and add an extra rinse cycle.
  - Clothing should be cotton or cotton-blend and avoidance of occlusive clothing is important.
  - Avoid temperatures resulting in sweating.
  - Shower and wash with a mild soap immediately after swimming in a pool to remove pool chemicals, immediately followed by application of moisturizer.
  - Nonsensitizing sunscreen should be used before sun exposure, and products developed for use on the face are often best tolerated by patients with AD.
  - Prolonged sun exposure can result in exacerbation due to evaporative losses and sweating.
- **When a specific antigen is identified that worsens AD, allergen avoidance can be effective.**
  - If a specific food is implicated in a controlled challenge, avoidance results in clinical improvement.[13]
  - 90% of the food allergens found to exacerbate AD that include milk, egg, peanut, soy, wheat, and fish.
  - **Extensive elimination diets are a bad idea.** Even patients with multiple positive allergy tests are rarely clinically sensitive to more than three foods on challenge.
  - Patients with dust mite allergen-specific IgE often demonstrate improvement in their AD after taking measures to reduce dust mite exposure.

Hydration
- Skin hydration is essential since atopic skin shows enhanced water loss and reduced water-binding capacity.
- An effective method for improving skin hydration is to soak skin for 10 minutes in warm water, then apply an occlusive agent within a few minutes to retain the absorbed water. For soaking of the face and neck, apply a warm wet washcloth.
- Bleach baths with one-half cup bleach per full bathtub have been recommended to reduce skin infections.[14]

- Moisturizers also have an important role in improving skin hydration.
  - Lotions have higher water content than creams, resulting in more drying of the skin due to an evaporative effect.
  - Because moisturizers should be applied **multiple times daily** on a long-term basis, cost is an obvious concern.
  - **Petroleum jelly** is an inexpensive option that is especially effective as an occlusive to seal in water after bathing.

Wet-Wrap Dressings
- These dressings work by cooling the skin, providing a barrier to scratching, and enhancing penetration of topical corticosteroids.[15]
- Wet-wrap dressings are most effective when covered with dry dressings or clothing and is often best tolerated at bedtime.

Phototherapy
- Ultraviolet (UV) light therapy can be useful for chronic recalcitrant AD.
- Some patients benefit from moderate amounts of natural sunlight.
- Photochemotherapy with oral methoxypsoralen followed by UV-A may be helpful in patients with severe AD who do not tolerate topical steroids.

COMPLICATIONS

- Eye:
  - **Atopic keratoconjunctivitis** is characterized by bilateral eye itching, burning, tearing, and mucoid discharge. It can result in visual impairment from corneal scarring.
  - **Keratoconus** is a conical corneal deformity due to persistent rubbing. Left untreated keratoconus may lead to formation of anterior subcapsular cataracts.
- Hand: Nonspecific **irritant hand dermatitis** is common in AD; irritated by repeated wetting.
- Infections:
  - AD confers an increased susceptibility to viruses, including herpes simplex virus (HSV), molluscum contagiosum, and human papilloma virus (HPV).
  - Patients are also at risk for superimposed dermatophytosis.
  - *S. aureus* colonizes the skin of >90% of patients with AD, compared to 5% of normal subjects. This can result in recurrent staphylococcal pustulosis but invasive *S. aureus* infections are rare.

REFERENCES

1. Boguniewicz M, Leung DY. Atopic Dermatitis. In: Adkinson N, et al., eds. *Middleton's Allergy: Principles and Practice.* 7th ed. Philadelphia, PA: Elsevier, 2009:1083–1103.
2. Illi S, von Mutius E, Lau S, et al. The natural course of atopic dermatitis from birth to age 7 years and the association with asthma. *J Allergy Clin Immunol.* 2004;113:925–931.
3. Sugiura H, Umemoto N, Deguchi H, et al. Prevalence of childhood and adolescent atopic dermatitis in a Japanese population: comparison with the disease frequency examined 20 years ago. *Acta Derm Venereol.* 1998;78:293–294.
4. Ong PY, Ohtake T, Brandt C, et al. Endogenous antimicrobial peptides and skin infections in atopic dermatitis. *N Engl J Med.* 2002;347:1151–1160.
5. Sampson HA, McCaskill CC. Food hypersensitivity and atopic dermatitis: evaluation of 113 patients. *J Pediatr.* 1985;107:669–675.

6. Irvine AD, McLean WH, Leung DY. Filaggrin mutations associated with skin and allergic diseases. *N Engl J Med.* 2011;365:1315–1327.
7. Hubiche T, Ged C, Benard A, et al. Analysis of SPINK 5, KLK 7 and FLG genotypes in a French atopic dermatitis cohort. *Acta Derm Venereol.* 2007;87:499–505.
8. Brandt EB, Sivagrasad U. Th2 cytokines and atopic dermatitis. *J Clin Cell Immunol.* 2011; 2:1–25.
9. Jariwala SP, Abrams E, Benson A, et al. The role of thymic stromal lymphopoietin in the immunopathogenesis of atopic dermatitis. *Clin Exp Allergy.* 2011;41:1515–1520.
10. Peserico A, Städtler G, Sebastian M, et al. Reduction of relapses of atopic dermatitis with methylprednisolone aceponate cream twice weekly in addition to maintenance treatment with emollient: a multicentre, randomized, double-blind, controlled study. *Br J Dermatol.* 2008;158:801–807.
11. Hung SH, Lin YRT, Chu CY, et al. Staphylococcus colonization in atopic dermatitis treated with fluticasone or tacrolimus with or without antibiotics. *Ann Allergy Asthma Immunol.* 2007;98:51–56.
12. Gollnick H, Kaufmann R, Stough D, et al. Pimecrolimus cream 1% in the long-term management of adult atopic dermatitis: prevention of flare progression. A randomized controlled trial. *Br J Dermatol.* 2008;158:1083–1093.
13. Schmitt J, Schäkel K, Schmitt N, et al. Systemic treatment of severe atopic eczema: a systemic review. *Acta Derm Venereol.* 2007;87:100–111.
14. Huang JT, Abrams M, Tlougan B, et al. Treatment of *Staphylococcus aureus* colonization in atopic dermatitis decreases disease severity. *Pediatrics.* 2009;123:e808–e814.
15. Devillers AC, Oranie AP. Efficacy and safety of 'wet-wrap' dressings as an intervention treatment in children with severe and/or refractory atopic dermatitis: a critical review of the literature. *Br J Dermatol.* 2006;154:579–585.

Allergic Contact Dermatitis

11

Olajumoke O. Fadugba

GENERAL PRINCIPLES

- Contact dermatitis is an eczematous rash that develops after the skin is in contact with a topical offending agent. **The agent may directly or indirectly cause injury to the skin.**
- There are two categories of contact dermatitis, which include irritant contact dermatitis (ICD) and allergic contact dermatitis (ACD).

Definition

- **ICD results from direct injury to the skin and is not immunologically mediated.** Typical agents that lead to this rash include acids, bases, and exposure to chronically wet environment, soaps and detergents.
- **ACD is an immunologically mediated reaction** that requires an initial exposure to a substance. The most common causative agents are plants of the *Rhus* genus (poison ivy, poison oak, poison sumac).

Epidemiology

- Prevalence of ACD in the general population is 20%.[1]
- Occupational ACD has a 12-month prevalence of 1,700 per 100,000 workers in one study.[2]

Pathophysiology

- ACD results from a type IV hypersensitivity reaction (see Chapter 2) that is mediated by a T-cell pathway. Unlike many allergic diseases, ACD elicits a T_H1 type of response.
- There are two phases, which include a sensitization phase and an elicitation phase.
- **Sensitization phase:**
  - Sensitization begins when a topical antigen comes into contact with the skin.
  - Typically molecules that are <500 Da result in ACD because the insulting agent must be small enough to penetrate the horny layer of the skin and enter into the stratum corneum.[3]
  - Once the antigen penetrates the skin, the antigen comes in contact with Langerhans cells or other antigen-presenting cells.
  - Langerhans cells are then drained by the lymphatic system to local lymph nodes where they become opposed to helper T lymphocytes.[3]
  - T cells then proliferate via clonal expansion and eventually memory T cells are created.
  - The production of memory T cells can take 4–7 days, and an individual can stay sensitized for several years.

- **Elicitation phase:**
  - The elicitation phase begins when patients are re-exposed to the allergen resulting in activation of local sensitized CD4+ T lymphocytes.
  - Several proinflammatory mediators are activated such as interleukin (IL)-1, IL-2, interferon (IFN)-γ leading to chemoattraction of macrophages, mast cells, basophils, and eosinophils to the area of exposure. This leads to the typical eczematous rash associated with contact dermatitis.

Risk Factors

- Patients who have a history of atopic dermatitis or ICD are at increased risk of developing ACD.
- Also, patients with ACD are at increased risk of developing ICD in their occupational environment.

DIAGNOSIS

Clinical Presentation

History

- The most common chief complaint of patient presenting with ACD is pruritus.
- Many patients develop an erythematous rash that progresses to papules after coming into contact with the allergen.
  - Symptoms typically develop 4–72 hours after exposure to the allergen.
  - The clinician should investigate over what course of time did the rash develop and/or change, has the rash occurred before, where has the rash occurred, if there is any improvement in the rash when the patient is on vacation or away from work/home.
- A thorough review of the patient's occupation, travel, social, and medical history is necessary to identify any possible exposures to common allergens. This should include any leisure activities the patient partakes.
- There are several allergens that commonly cause ACD and include the following: **Poison ivy, nickel, fragrances, latex, paraphenylenediamine** (found in dyes and rubber), and **neomycin.**[2]

Physical Examination

- ACD can occur on any part of the body.
  - Areas of thin skin such as eyes, neck, and genitalia are the most susceptible to ACD.
  - The areas that are most resistant to sensitization include the palms, soles, and scalp.
  - The most characteristic feature of the rash is to **occur at the site of contact** with the allergen.
- The appearance of the rash depends on the time of presentation.
  - Initially, an area or erythema develops followed by eruption of papules or vesicles.
  - Eventually the vesicle will involute and crusting and scaling will develop.
  - Patients that are chronically exposed to an allergy develop lichenification, painful fissuring, and thickening of the skin.
- Distribution and pattern of the rash is very important to note on physical examination as this provides clues as to which allergen contributes to the rash.
  - Eczematous rash localized to earlobes or wrist indicates possible nickel allergy found in jewelry.

○ Linear patterned rashes are usually caused by poison ivy.

○ Involvement of head and neck suggest possible cosmetics, hair dyes, or relaxers.

○ If the rash is only found under areas where clothes are in contact suggests a reaction to allergen found in textiles.

○ Undergarments and shoes are made of rubber products and patients will have rashes located in these respective areas.

• Systemically administered medications can cross react with topically applied medications leading to generalized ACD.

Differential Diagnosis

• Other conditions that can have an appearance similar to ACD include:[2]

○ Seborrheic dermatitis.

○ Nummular eczema.

○ Dyshidrotic eczema.

○ Atopic dermatitis (see Chapter 10).

○ ICD.

Diagnostic Testing

• *Patch testing* can aid in the diagnosis of ACD.

○ Patch testing involves placing patch(es) containing a small amount of the allergen on the patient's back.

▪ Commercially available preparations for patch testing that use amounts of allergen considered to be nonirritating.

○ After a minimum of 48 hours and up to 7 days, the patch is removed and the degree of inflammation (if any) is assessed.

○ A positive patch test is one where there is evidence of inflammation at the patch site and indicates the patient has been sensitized to the allergen.

○ Results of a patch test should be interpreted in the setting of the patient's history.

• Often, the suspected offending agent is not available for patch testing. In these cases, elimination of the trigger from the patient's environment can be diagnostic and therapeutic.

TREATMENT

• The **first-line** therapy of ACD is to identify and avoid the triggering allergen.

• There are several topical medications that are used in order to treat aggravating symptoms.

Medications

• Localized acute ACD on the body can be treated with topical corticosteroid creams such as triamcinolone or clobetastol.

○ Cream-based topical steroids are preferable as they have a more drying effect than ointments.[3]

○ Caution should be used when using topical steroids as they can thin skin.

• Systemic steroids should be considered in severe cases of ACD that involve large areas of skin.

• Oral antihistaminic medications maybe needed during the first days of starting either systemic or topical steroids, especially for patients having difficulty sleeping secondary to severe pruritis.

- All these medications are symptomatic treatments. To prevent the rash from occurring, the patient should avoid triggering agents.

Other Nonpharmacologic Therapies

- Cool, moist compresses can provide a soothing effect to areas with weepy lesions.[3]
- Oatmeal baths can help in symptomatic control of ACD affecting large areas of skin.[3]
- Drying antipruritic lotions such as calamine lotion can be used on localized ACD.
- Topical antihistamines and anesthetics should be avoided as these agents can lead to sensitization.

REFERENCES

1. Gotthard C, Anderson EA. New aspects in allergic contact dermatitis. *Curr Opin Allergy Clin Immunol.* 2008;8:428–432.
2. Usatine RP, Riojas M. Diagnosis and management of contact dermatitis. *Am Fam Physician.* 2010;82:249–255.
3. Rietschel RP, Fowler JF, eds. *Fischer's Contact Dermatitis,* 6th ed. Lewiston, NY: BC Decker Inc, 2008.

Ocular Allergic Disease

12

Gregg J. Berdy and Susan S. Berdy

GENERAL PRINCIPLES

Ocular allergic diseases can be considered a spectrum of diseases ranging from mild itching and redness associated with seasonal allergic conjunctivitis to severe blinding sequelae secondary to atopic keratoconjunctivitis.

Definition

Immunoglobulin E (IgE)-mediated inflammation of the conjunctivae, clear membrane that covers the sclera and lines the eyelids.

Classification

Ocular allergic conditions may be classified as follows:[1]
* Seasonal allergic conjunctivitis (SAC)
* Vernal keratoconjunctivitis (VKC), palpebral or limbal
* Atopic keratoconjunctivitis (AKC)
* Giant papillary conjunctivitis (GPC)

Epidemiology

Approximately 20–30% (60–90 million people) of the population of the United States suffer from ocular allergic diseases.

Etiology

Genetic predisposition for atopy and formation of specific IgE after exposure to environmental allergens.

Pathophysiology

* SAC is the prototype of the group of diseases that begins as an **antigen–IgE antibody interaction on the surface of the conjunctival mast cells.**[2]
* The allergen binds two separate IgE molecules, creating a dimer formation (cross-linking) that initiates the chain of reactions on the mast cell plasma membrane.
* Cross-linking of the IgE causes the release of preformed mediators (e.g., histamine) and newly formed mediators produced via metabolism of arachidonic acid (AA).
* Metabolism of AA produces **prostaglandins** via the cyclooxygenase pathway and **leukotrienes** via the lipoxygenase pathway.
* Conjunctival surface contains both H1 and H2 histamine receptors.
  ○ Histamine binding to the H1 receptor results in symptoms of ocular **itching.**
  ○ Histamine binding to the H2 receptors produces **vasodilation of conjunctival vessels.**

- Other mediators:
  - Eosinophils release **major basic protein** (MBP) that has been demonstrated to cause epithelial toxicity.
  - Lymphocytes release **interleukins** that is involved in further recruitment of inflammatory cells and their release of inflammatory mediators.
  - **T-lymphocyte abnormalities** have been demonstrated in AKC (TH1) and VKC (TH2).

Risk Factors

- SAC:
  - Family history of atopy.
  - 70% of patients have an associated atopic disease, such as allergic rhinitis, asthma, or atopic dermatitis.
- VKC:
  - Usually seen in children aged 4–18 years.
  - Boys are affected more frequently than girls.
  - Affected individuals usually live in warm to hot windy climate.
  - Strong family history of atopic disease.
- AKC:
  - Chronic disease usually seen in patients aged 50–60 years.
  - Long history of eczema or atopic dermatitis.
- GPC:
  - Chronic inflammatory disorder.
  - Exogenous materials causing chronic inflammation of the upper tarsal conjunctival surface.
  - Most cases are secondary to **soft contact lens wear,** but ocular prostheses and nylon sutures used in ophthalmic surgical procedures may be an etiologic agent.

Associated Conditions

- Allergic rhinitis
- Asthma

DIAGNOSIS

- Diagnosis can be made by taking a careful history and performing epicutaneous skin testing with environmental allergens to either confirm or exclude the presence of allergic sensitization.
- Physical examination of the eyes, including assessment of the eyelids, conjunctivae and quality of tears that are formed, and slit lamp examination where warranted.

Clinical Presentation

History
- SAC:
  - Bilateral red, itching eyes associated with tearing and burning.
  - Occasionally unilateral response may occur when there has been hand-to-eye contact with allergen (e.g., cat dander).

- VKC:
  - Typically young boy will present with marked itching associated with a stringy, ropy mucus discharge.
  - Severe cases may be associated with photophobia, pain, and decreased visual acuity.
- AKC: Chronic year-round itching; associated with burning, light sensitivity, tearing, and chronic redness of the eyes.
- GPC:
  - Patients complain of chronic irritation, redness, and itching.
  - Decreased wearing time of contact lenses.
  - Increasing mucus discharge associated with pain, tearing, and conjunctival redness.

Physical Examination
- SAC:
  - Edematous and erythematous periocular tissues.
  - Conjunctiva with mild to moderate chemosis with mucous discharge in the tear film.
  - Cornea is rarely involved.
- VKC:
  - Edematous and ptotic upper eyelid.
  - Corneal examination may reveal superficial infiltrates and in severe cases **shield ulcers**, which are epithelial defects with plaque-like deposition of material at the base, centrally located just above the visual axis.
  - Palpebral VKC:
    - Upper tarsal surface develops large raised **cobblestone papillae**, which are pathognomonic of the disease.
    - Papillae appear injected and commonly have mucus strands running in the crevices.
  - Limbal VKC:
    - Lid eversion reveals Horner's points–Tranta's dots.
    - These are aggregations of eosinophils and grossly appear as gelatinous elevations with whitish inclusions located at the limbus.
- AKC:
  - Eczematoid changes of the upper and lower eyelids, induration, erythema, and scaling.
  - Slit lamp examination reveals marked plugging of the meibomian gland orifices with purulent secretions and a concurrent poor precorneal tear film.
  - Bulbar conjunctiva may show mild to moderate injection and changes consistent with keratoconjunctivitis sicca (KCS) (dry eye).
  - Severe cases may result in conjunctival subepithelial fibrosis and **symblepharon** formation.
  - Tarsal conjunctival surfaces usually reveal mild to moderate injection.
  - Corneal involvement in AKC may vary according to the severity of disease.
    - In mild forms the cornea may show minimal punctate staining with fluorescein dye.
    - Severe cases demonstrate marked surface irregularity with epithelial desiccation associated with corneal neovascularization, keratinization, and scarring.
- GPC:
  - Examination may reveal minimal pathology.
  - Hyperemia and **giant papillae** may develop with chronic trauma to the upper tarsal conjunctival surfaces.

○ Papillae are result of chronic collagen deposition and tend to be more uniformly distributed, smaller, and flatter in appearance than those seen in the cobblestone appearance of patients with VKC.

○ With disease progression, cornea may show diffuse punctate keratitis or even corneal epithelial abrasions.

Differential Diagnosis

- Viral conjunctivitis:[3]
  ○ Usually characterized by an acute onset of a unilateral red eye associated with preauricular lymph node.
  ○ Patients complain of matting of the eyelids with clear to mucopurulent discharge.
  ○ Examination of the tarsal conjunctivae reveals a follicular appearance.
  ○ Infection often spreads to the opposite eye 3–9 days later.
  ○ May have concurrent upper respiratory infection.
- Bacterial conjunctivitis:
  ○ Usually characterized by an acute onset of a unilateral or bilateral red eye associated with eyelid erythema.
  ○ Patients complain of matting of the eyelashes with yellow to green purulent discharge.
  ○ Examination of the tarsal conjunctivae reveals a papillary appearance.
- Chlamydial conjunctivitis:
  ○ Usually characterized by an indolent, chronic onset of at least 6 weeks of a unilateral or bilateral mildly red eye.
  ○ Examination of the tarsal conjunctivae reveals a mixed follicular and papillary appearance.
- Noninfectious:
  ○ Contact dermatitis.
  ○ Drug-induced allergic contact dermatitis.
  ○ KCS, dry eye syndrome.
  ○ Meibomian gland dysfunction (MGD), blepharitis.

TREATMENT

- Identify and remove the offending allergen.
- Prevent circulating allergens from interacting with conjunctival mast cells.
  ○ Diluting antigen load with tear substitutes.
  ○ Immunotherapy.
- Suppress cellular and extracellular inflammation with concomitant redness (vascular dilation) and chemosis (edema) using vasoconstrictor agents, nonsteroidal antiinflammatory drugs (NSAIDs), and steroidal agents.
- Decrease and prevent itching associated redness by using mast cell stabilizer/antihistamine dual acting agents (see Table 12-1).[4]
- Decrease itching by using H1-receptor antihistamines.
- **For GPC specifically, discontinue the use of contact lens wear for 4–6 weeks.**

MEDICATIONS

Seasonal Allergic Conjunctivitis
First Line
- Topical mast cell stabilizers/antihistamine dual acting agents.

TABLE 12-1	ALLERGIC CONJUNCTIVITIS MEDICATIONS

Combination mast cell stabilizer/H1-receptor antagonist:

Olopatadine
Bepotastine
Alcaftadine
Azelastine
Epinastine

Selective H1-receptor antagonists:

Levocabastine
Emedastine

Mast cell stabilizers:

Lodoxamide tromethamine
Nedocromil
Pemirolast
Cromolyn

NSAIDs:

Ketorolac

Topical steroid:

Loteprednol

NSAIDs, nonsteroidal antiinflammatory drugs.

Second Line
- Topical selective H1-receptor antagonists.
- Topical mast cell stabilizers.
- Topical NSAIDs.
- Topical antihistamine/decongestants (over the counter).

Third Line
- Topical steroid eye drops.
- Systemic corticosteroids (rarely needed).

Vernal Keratoconjunctivitis
First Line
- Topical mast cell stabilizers/antihistamine dual acting agents.
- Topical mast cell stabilizers.

Second Line
- Topical selective H1-receptor antagonists.
- Topical NSAIDs.
- Topical steroids.

Third Line
- Systemic antihistamines.
- Occasionally requires short pulses of systemic steroids.

Atopic Keratoconjunctivitis

First Line
- Topical mast cell stabilizers/antihistamine dual acting agents.
- Topical steroids.
- Topical cyclosporine A.
- Topical antibiotic drops or ointments if corneal abrasion or keratitis is present.
- Tear replacements, consider preservative free.

Second Line
- Systemic antibiotics:
  - Doxycycline 100 mg bid.
  - Minocycline 100 mg bid.
- Systemic antihistamines.
- Eyelid scrubs with baby shampoo.

Giant Papillary Conjunctivitis

First Line
- Topical mast cell stabilizers/antihistamine dual acting agents.
- Topical mast cell stabilizers.
- Topical NSAIDs.

Second Line
- Topical steroids.

Atopic Contact Dermatitis of Eyelids

First Line
- Topical 1% hydrocortisone cream to eyelid skin.
- Topical calcineurin inhibitors to eyelid skin (e.g., pimecrolimus and tacrolimus ointment).
- Topical unscented lubricant cream to eyelid skin.
- Eucerin cream.

Second Line
- If conjunctival involvement exists:
  - Topical mast cell stabilizers/antihistamine dual acting agents.
  - Topical NSAIDs.
  - Topical steroids.

Other Treatments
- Identification and avoidance of allergens.
- Cool compresses.
- Irrigation with artificial tears.
- Allergy immunotherapy.

SPECIAL CONSIDERATIONS

- Patients being treated with topical steroid drops should have close ophthalmology monitoring to watch for increased intraocular pressure, corneal ulcers, and cataracts.
- The most important aspects of treating ocular allergic disease are a careful history taking and making a differential diagnosis.
- Rule out other causes of red, itchy eyes.

REFERRAL

- Allergy/immunology evaluation to confirm or exclude IgE-mediated disease.
- Ophthalmology evaluation.

REFERENCES

1. Berdy GJ, Berdy SS. Ocular allergic disorders: disease entities and differential diagnoses. *Curr Allergy Asthma Rep.* 2009;9:297–303.
2. Ono SJ, Abelson MB. Allergic conjunctivitis: update on pathophysiology and prospects for future treatment. *J Allergy Clin Immunol.* 2005;115:118–122.
3. Bielory L. Differential diagnoses of conjunctivitis for clinical allergist immunologists. *Ann Allergy Asthma Immunol.* 2007;98:105–115.
4. Berdy GJ, Spangler DL, Bensch G, et al. A comparison of the relative efficacy and clinical performance of olopatadine hydrochloride 0.1% ophthalmic solution and ketotifen fumarate 0.025% ophthalmic solution in the conjunctival antigen challenge model. *Clin Ther.* 2000;22:826–833.

Anaphylaxis

13

Sydney Leibel

GENERAL PRINCIPLES

- Anaphylaxis is a severe, life-threatening multi-organ hypersensitivity reaction of rapid onset.[1]
- **Anaphylaxis is a medical emergency.**

Epidemiology

- **There are an estimated 700 fatal anaphylactic reactions per year in the United States.**
- In many of these cases, epinephrine was unfortunately never administered.
- Incidence of 50–200 episodes/100,000 person/years. Lifetime prevalence of 0.05–2%.[2]
- True incidence is unknown due to under-diagnosis and under-reporting.

Etiology

- Broadly, the causes of anaphylaxis are divided into immunoglobulin E (IgE)-dependent and IgE-independent (formerly called anaphylactoid) mechanisms.[3]
- IgE-mediated mechanisms include:
  - Medications (Chap. 14)
  - Insect bites and stings (Chap. 15)
  - Foods (Chap. 16)
  - Latex (Chap. 17)
  - Allergen immunotherapy (Chap. 21)
  - Others (e.g., seminal fluid)
- IgE-independent mechanisms:
  - Radiocontrast medium (Chap. 14)
  - Opioid medications
  - Vancomycin
  - Aspirin/nonsteroidal antiinflammatory drugs (NSAIDs)
  - Scombroid fish poisoning
  - Blood products (e.g., in immunoglobulin A-deficient patients)
  - Idiopathic
- Mastocytosis can also manifest with anaphylaxis.

Pathophysiology

- Anaphylaxis is a type I or immediate hypersensitivity reaction (Chap. 2).
- It is elicited by the **cross-linking of allergen-specific IgE bound to the surface of mast cells and basophils by allergens** leading to the release of preformed and synthesized chemical mediators.[4]

- Cross-linking promotes the **immediate (5–30 minute) release of granule-associated preformed mediators:** Histamine, tryptase, carboxypeptidase A, chymase, and proteoglycans.
- In addition, there is **synthesis of newly generated mediators:** Prostaglandins, leukotrienes, sphingosine 1-phosphate, platelet activating factor, and cytokines interleukin (IL) 6, IL33, and tumor necrosis factor (TNF)-α over a period of **2–6 hours.**
- Other mechanisms include complement breakdown products (C3a, C4a, C5a) and the contact system activation bradykinin.

Risk Factors

- History of prior anaphylaxis.
- Parenteral exposure to antigen is associated with higher risk of anaphylaxis compared to ingestion.
- Intermittent exposure to antigen.
- Large dose exposure.
- In children <15 years old, males are at higher risk. For adults, females are at higher risk.
- Adults are at higher risk for anaphylaxis due to penicillin and *Hymenoptera,* whereas children are at higher risk for food-induced anaphylaxis.
- Atopy does not appear to increase the risk of anaphylaxis, but it may place an individual at risk for more severe expressions of anaphylaxis, including death.
- β-blocker therapy places an individual at risk for a more severe anaphylaxis reaction and may make resuscitation more difficult.

DIAGNOSIS

Clinical Presentation

- The clinical manifestations of anaphylaxis are highly variable. Signs and symptoms include any combination of the following (listed in order of frequency) ranging from a mild to life-threatening severe reaction[5]:
  - **Dermatologic** (80–90%): Flushing, urticaria, angioedema, and pruritus.
  - **Respiratory** (up to 70%): Rhinorrhea/sneezing, cough, choking, stridor, wheeze, bronchospasm, and laryngeal edema.
  - **Cardiovascular** (up to 45%): Hypotension, tachycardia, arrhythmia, myocardial infarction, and syncope.
  - **Gastrointestinal/genitourinary** (up to 45%): Abdominal or uterine cramping, diarrhea, nausea, and vomiting.
- Although cutaneous symptoms are common in anaphylaxis, they are not necessary to confirm the diagnosis. Similarly hypotension may not be present (Table 13-1).[1]
- Onset of symptoms is typically within minutes of exposure to antigen, although in rare circumstances it can be delayed for hours.
- **Median time to symptoms/cardiovascular collapse is 30 minutes for food exposure and 5 minutes for parenterally administered agents.**[6]
- A diagnosis of anaphylaxis should be considered when there is an acute onset of symptoms in two organ systems, especially in the setting of an exposure to a possible provoking antigen.
- If the patient has a known allergy to a particular allergen, hypotension after exposure to that antigen is enough to make the diagnosis of anaphylaxis.
- **A delayed reaction can occur in some individuals (biphasic reaction),** leading to recurrence of symptoms 4–8 hours after the initial event.

TABLE 13-1	CLINICAL DIAGNOSIS OF ANAPHYLAXIS

Anaphylaxis is likely when one of the three criteria occurs:

1. Acute skin and/or mucosal symptoms (e.g., hives, pruritus, flushing, lip/tongue/uvula swelling) and one of the following:
   - Respiratory symptoms (e.g., wheezing, stridor, shortness of breath, hypoxia)
   - Hypotension or associated end-organ dysfunction (e.g., hypotonia, syncope, incontinence)
2. Exposure to probable allergen for the patient and ≥2 of the following:
   - Skin-mucosal tissue involvement
   - Respiratory symptoms
   - Hypotension or end-organ dysfunction
   - Persistent gastrointestinal symptoms (e.g., emesis, abdominal pain)
3. Decreased blood pressure after exposure to known allergen for the patient
   - Adults: Systolic blood pressure <90 mm Hg or >30% decrease
   - Infants and children: Hypotension for age or >30% decrease in systolic blood pressure

Adapted from: Sampson HA, Muñoz-Furlong A, Campbell RL, et al. Second symposium on the definition and management of anaphylaxis: Summary report—Second National Institute of Allergy and Infectious Disease/Food Allergy and Anaphylaxis Network symposium. *J Allergy Clin Immunol* 2006;117:391–397.

- **Protracted anaphylaxis** requiring many hours of active resuscitation occurs in as many as 28% of patients.[7]
- Risk factors for prolonged anaphylaxis are oral ingestion of the allergen, onset of symptoms more than 30 minutes after exposure to the stimulus, and lack of epinephrine administration.
- **Recurrent episodes** of anaphylaxis without a known cause warrant consideration of other diagnoses. **Systemic mastocytosis** (Chapter 19) can present with recurrent anaphylaxis. Total tryptase will be elevated persistently even when patient is asymptomatic.
- If all other diagnoses are excluded, **idiopathic anaphylaxis** should be considered.
  - Idiopathic anaphylaxis is a **diagnosis of exclusion** with no causative factor identified and thought to be the result of **nonimmunologic mast cell activation.**
  - Clinical presentation and treatment are the same as for anaphylaxis due to known allergens.
  - Patients who have more than six episodes per year may be considered for placement on maintenance prednisone therapy.

Differential Diagnosis

The differential diagnosis of anaphylaxis is presented in Table 13-2.

Diagnostic Testing

Laboratories

- If the diagnosis of anaphylaxis is in question, it is possible to measure a serum β-tryptase level after patient stabilization. Studies have shown that increased levels of β-tryptase correspond to acute mediator release.

TABLE 13-2	DIFFERENTIAL DIAGNOSIS OF ANAPHYLAXIS

Vasovagal reaction
Other causes of angioedema (e.g., angiotensin converting enzyme inhibitors, hereditary angioedema)
Arrhythmias
Cardiogenic shock
Sepsis syndrome
Hypoglycemia
Serotonin syndrome/carcinoid syndrome
Adrenal insufficiency
Panic disorder

- In the case of an insect sting anaphylaxis, β-tryptase blood levels are maximal 15–120 minutes after anaphylaxis and decline with a half-life of 1.5–2.5 hours.[8]
- β-tryptase levels are measurable for up to 8 hours after a putative anaphylactic reaction.
- Levels may not be elevated in food-mediated anaphylaxis.

Diagnostic Procedures

Skin Testing

- Patients are often referred to an allergist after an episode of presumed anaphylaxis. If a careful history unveils the causative agent, confirmation can be performed with skin testing, *in vitro,* or challenge testing (Chap. 8).
- However, **skin tests are not reliable for up to 4–6 weeks after an episode of anaphylaxis due to expended mast cell degranulation.**
- A single episode of anaphylaxis with no obvious causative antigen by history does not warrant random skin testing or *in vitro* testing.
- *In vitro* antigen-specific IgE can be tested immediately after an episode of anaphylaxis but is less sensitive than skin testing.

TREATMENT

- Regardless of severity, all anaphylactic episodes deserve treatment and observation, as any mild reaction can rapidly degrade into a more serious reaction.
- For **acute treatment,** the initial assessment is paramount for prompt recognition of symptoms and immediate institution of treatment (see Fig. 13-1).
- The **first line of therapy is epinephrine,** and it should be administered immediately (Fig. 13-1).[9]
- The patient may require cardiopulmonary resuscitation to support the airway, maintain adequate oxygenation and circulation.
- Treatment also includes long-term risk management.
  ○ Prepare for emergencies with an **anaphylaxis emergency action plan** (see www.aaaai.org), **autoinjector, and medical identification.**
  ○ Take steps to reduce long-term risk: Assess and treat comorbidities (asthma, cardiovascular disease, mastocytosis, and others); assess for comedications such as nonselective β-blockers; and avoid known allergens (for more information, see www.foodallergy.org, www.latexallergyresources.org, and www.aaaai.org).

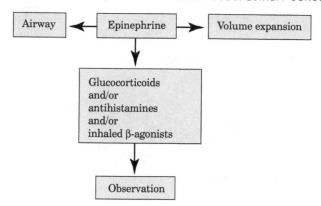

FIGURE 13-1 Management of anaphylaxis.

○ Consider allergen-specific and allergen non-specific immunomodulation. Allergen-specific includes immunotherapy with insect venom and desensitization to β-lactam antibiotics, NSAIDs, and others. For idiopathic anaphylaxis consider glucocorticoid treatment.

Medications

Epinephrine

- **Epinephrine is the only known medication that can prevent or reverse obstruction to airflow in upper and lower airways and prevent or reverse cardiovascular collapse.**
- Failure to inject epinephrine in a timely manner is reported to contribute to fatality.[6]
- There are no absolute contraindications to its use.
- **It should be administered immediately using a dose of 0.3–0.5 mg IM** (0.3–0.5 mL of a 1:1,000 solution) in the anterolateral thigh preferentially or upper extremity (deltoid).
- Epinephrine dose may be repeated at 5-minute intervals as needed.
- Smaller doses may be needed in the elderly (0.2 mg).
- In children, the dose is 0.01 mg/kg (1:1,000) IM to a maximum of 0.5 mg with repeated doses every 5 minutes as needed.
- Larger doses may be needed in patients receiving β-blockers. **Glucagon** (1–2 mg IV push) may be needed in these patients.
- Administration via central line (3–5 mL of **1:10,000 solution**) or through endotracheal tube (3–5 mL of a **1:10,000 solution diluted in 10 mL normal saline**) may be necessary in cases of severe hypotension or respiratory failure.
- A continuous infusion of 1:10,000 epinephrine may be necessary in patients with protracted symptoms.
  ○ **Potential risks of IV epinephrine include myocardial ischemia and infarction, arrhythmias, and hypertensive crisis.**
  ○ A bolus of 100 μg/70 kg over a period of 5–10 minutes may be given (1:10,000 concentration). A continuous infusion of 1–5 μg/min/70 kg is usually sufficient to maintain systemic perfusion.

Glucocorticosteroids

- **Glucocorticosteroids do not have an immediate effect, and their use is currently considered ancillary.**
- Glucocorticosteroids have the theoretical ability to prevent a relapse of symptoms based on management of acute asthma and the abrogation of the late-phase response. However, the ability to prevent an anaphylactic biphasic reaction has not been proven in a controlled study.

Antihistamines

- **Antihistamines will also not have an immediate effect but may shorten the duration of symptoms.**
- **Diphenhydramine** can be administered IV (25–100 mg over 5–10 minutes), IM, or PO. It can be given every 6 hours for 24–48 hours after the reaction.
- **H2 antagonists** (i.e., ranitidine, cimetidine) may also be added.[10]

Bronchodilators

- **In patients with asthma who are undergoing anaphylaxis-associated wheezing, epinephrine remains the first line of therapy.**
- However, if wheezing persists, bronchodilators such as albuterol (nebulized every 20 minutes or continuously) or theophylline may be considered.

Nonpharmacologic Therapies
Airway Management

- Airway management may require endotracheal intubation if marked stridor or respiratory failure occurs.
- **Racemic epinephrine** may be useful in treating laryngeal edema.
- **If laryngeal edema is severe and not immediately responsive to epinephrine, consider cricothyroidotomy or tracheotomy.**

Volume Expansion

- Significant third spacing of fluid may occur in anaphylaxis and the intravascular volume may decrease by up to 50%.
- Volume expansion with IV fluids, beginning with a 500–1,000 mL bolus, should be titrated to blood pressure and urine output.
- Colloid solutions, such as albumin, may be beneficial in cases of refractory hypotension or shock. The risk–benefit profile of each solution should be carefully weighed, as albumin may precipitate pulmonary edema and is rather costly.

Observation

- Patients with mild reactions limited to flushing, urticaria, angioedema, cramping, or mild bronchospasm should be monitored in the emergency department for a minimum of 6–8 hours for possible biphasic reaction.
- All other reactions warrant admission to the hospital for 24-hour observation.

Prevention

- Secondary prevention is predicated on **identification and avoidance of the inciting agent.**
- Accidental ingestion of allergic foods in the form of condiments and prepared foods is a well-known hazard, particularly for food-allergic children (Chap. 16).
- **If a known trigger is identified, a comprehensive avoidance strategy and action plan should be provided to the patient.**

- Medical identification (i.e., bracelet) may help healthcare professionals recognize a patient with a known history of anaphylaxis promptly.
- **Patients with a history of anaphylaxis due to food or** *Hymenoptera* **sting should carry self-administered epinephrine.**
- **Desensitization** in the case of certain drugs or immunotherapy in the case of venom (highly efficacious 95–98%) should be considered if future exposure to putative agent is unavoidable.

REFERENCES

1. Sampson HA, Muñoz-Furlong A, Campbell RL, et al. Second symposium on the definition and management of anaphylaxis: Summary report—Second National Institute of Allergy and Infectious Disease/Food Allergy and Anaphylaxis Network symposium. *J Allergy Clin Immunol* 2006;117:391–397.
2. Lieberman P, Camargo CA Jr, Bohlke K, et al. Epidemiology of anaphylaxis: findings of the American College of Allergy Asthma and Immunology Epidemiology of Anaphylaxis Working Group. *Ann Allergy Asthma Immunol* 2006;97:596–602.
3. Decker WW, Campbell RL, Manivannan V, et al. The etiology and incidence of anaphylaxis in Rochester, Minnesota: a report from the Rochester Epidemiology Project. *J Allergy Clin Immunol* 2008;122:1161–1165.
4. Peavy RD, Metcalfe DD. Understanding the mechanisms of anaphylaxis. *Curr Opin Allergy Clin Immunol* 2008;8:310–315.
5. Lieberman PL. Anaphylaxis. In: Adkinson NF, Bochner BS, Busse WW, et al., eds. *Middleton's Allergy Principles and Practice,* 7th ed. Philadelphia, PA: Elsevier Inc., 2009: 1027–1049.
6. Pumphrey RS. Lessons for management of anaphylaxis from a study of fatal reactions. *Clin Exp Allergy* 2000;30:1144–1150.
7. Stark BJ, Sullivan TJ. Biphasic and protracted anaphylaxis. *J Allergy Clin Immunol* 1986; 78:76–83.
8. Schwartz LB, Irani AA. Serum tryptase and the laboratory diagnosis of mastocytosis. *Hematol Oncol Clin North Am* 2000;14:641–657.
9. Simons FE. Anaphylaxis. *J Allergy Clin Immunol* 2008;121:S402–S407.
10. Ring J, Behrendt H. H1- and H2-antagonists in allergic and pseudoallergic diseases. *Clin Exp Allergy* 1990;20:43–49.

Drug Allergy and Desensitization

Jennifer M. Welch

GENERAL PRINCIPLES

Definition

- A drug allergy or hypersensitivity is a type of adverse drug reaction (ADR).
- An **ADR** is an undesired or unintended response that occurs when a drug is given for the appropriate purpose.
- Hypersensitivity should be used to describe **objectively reproducible symptoms or signs initiated by exposure to a defined stimulus at a dose tolerated by normal persons.**[1]
- **Allergy is a hypersensitivity reaction initiated by specific immunologic mechanisms.**[1] This can refer to immunoglobulin E (IgE)- or T-cell–mediated reactions.

Classification

- ADRs can be divided into two groups: Predictable adverse reactions and unpredictable adverse reactions.
- **Predictable adverse reactions are the most common and are often dose-dependent and related to the pharmacokinetics of the drug.** Examples are over dosage, known side effects (e.g., nausea with codeine), indirect effects (e.g., *Clostridium difficile* infection resulting from clindamycin administration for a skin infection), and drug–drug interactions.
- **Unpredictable adverse reactions are usually dose-independent and unrelated to the drug's pharmacokinetics.**
- Immune-mediated adverse reactions can be from various mechanisms. They usually occur upon re-exposure to the offending drug.
- Pseudoallergic reactions, formerly called anaphylactoid reactions, are caused by IgE-independent degranulation of mast cells.

Epidemiology

- A meta-analysis from studies conducted in the United States from 1966 to 1996 showed 15.1% of hospitalized patients experienced an ADR with an incidence of 3.1–6.2% of hospital admissions due to ADRs.[2]
- Overall mortality incidence from ADRs ranged from 0.14 to 0.32%.[3]
- Allergic drug reactions account for 6–10% of all observed ADRs. The risk for an allergic reaction is about 1–3% for most drugs. It is estimated that about 5% of adults may be allergic to one or more drugs.[4]

Pathophysiology

- High molecular weight (HMW) drugs, usually >4,000 Da, are large enough to elicit an immune response without interacting with other molecules.

- Low molecular weight (LMW) drugs, usually <1,000 Da, can form covalent bonds with a carrier protein, which can then elicit an immune response. This drug–protein formation is also known as the **hapten–carrier complex.**
- In some cases, the metabolite of a parent drug creates the immune response as it binds to another protein. The parent drug is referred to as a prohapten.
- A newer concept called p-i (pharmacologic interactions of drugs with immune receptors) concept states that a drug which cannot covalently bind to another protein can still elicit an immune response. This is achieved by activating T cells through van der Waals interactions with T-cell receptors or major histocompatibility complexes (MHCs).[5]
- **Immune-mediated drug reactions occur because an immune response is mounted against either drug or hapten–carrier.**
- The different immunologic mechanisms for a drug allergy are shown in the Gell and Coombs classification of hypersensitivity as explained in Chapter 2.
  - **Type I** reaction: IgE-mediated and immediate onset. Presents as anaphylaxis, urticaria, angioedema, asthma, and rhinitis.
  - **Type II** reaction: IgG antibody-mediated resulting in cytotoxic destruction of cells; delayed onset. Includes immune cytopenias.
  - **Type III** reaction: IgG:antigen complexes with complement activation. Onset delayed >1 week after drug exposure. Presents as serum sickness, vasculitis, or drug fever.
  - **Type IV** reaction: T-cell–mediated and delayed onset. Divided into four subtypes. Presents as contact dermatitis and various exanthems.
- Anaphylactoid or "pseudoallergic" reaction is not IgE mediated but results in the activation of macrophages and basophils. It is clinically indistinguishable from anaphylactic reactions.

Risk Factors

Drug Factors

- Size and structure: HMW drugs and the ability of a drug or its metabolite to bind to carrier proteins make it more immunogenic.
- Route of exposure: Cutaneous administration is the most immunogenic.[6] Penicillin (PCN) is no longer available topically due to this reason. Once sensitized, parental administration is associated more with anaphylaxis than oral administration.
- Dose, duration, and frequency: Increases in these three factors are more likely to elicit an immune response than in a smaller dose, for a short duration, and longer interval between therapy.

Patient-related Factors

- Age and gender: Women are affected more frequently than men.
- Genetic factors:
  - Atopy: Patients with a history of asthma, allergic rhinitis, or atopic dermatitis are not at increased risk for developing a drug reaction as compared to the general public. However, they may be at an increased risk to develop pseudoallergic reactions, in particular with radiocontrast media (RCM).[7]
  - Acetylators: A person who is a slow acetylator is at increased risk for ADR, such as developing drug-induced lupus (DIL) with hydralazine or procainamide.
  - Human leukocyte antigen (HLA) type: There have been numerous studies demonstrating certain HLA genes associated with increased risk of drug allergy. For

example, HLA-B*5701 is associated with a hypersensitivity reaction to abacavir.[8] Patients are now screened for this gene before initiating abacavir for treatment of HIV.
○ Family history of multiple drug allergies.
○ Prior drug reactions.
○ Coexisting medical illness: Some medical conditions, especially infections, predispose to an increased risk for ADRs.
  ■ Trimethoprim-sulfamethoxazole (TMP-SMX) hypersensitivity occurs in 5% of HIV-negative patients and in 60% of patients with HIV.[9]
  ■ In the setting of Epstein–Barr viral infection, administration of ampicillin produces a nearly universal maculopapular rash.[10]
○ Concurrent medial therapy: Patients treated with β-blocking agents may be diagnosed with an allergic reaction later into the reaction. β-blockade can impede treatment.

Prevention

• Prevention is vital to reduce the incidence of allergic drug reactions.
• It is important to only prescribe medications that are clinically essential.
• Minimizing polypharmacy also decreases the incidence of allergic drug reactions.
• If an allergy to a drug is in question, use skin testing where possible to further evaluate.
• A graded challenge will help to further delineate if the drug can be safely used at a therapeutic dose.
• Patients who have had an allergic drug reaction should be informed of the reaction and how to avoid further exposure, including the drug and any agents that may cross-react. The patient may carry a card or medical alert bracelet.
• Patients that require retreatment with the same drug or class of drugs have the following options:
  ○ **Administer an alternative:** This requires understanding the structure of the offending agent and the alternative drug.
  ○ **Administer a potentially cross-reactive drug under close medical supervision.** Skin testing may be performed, if available and reliable, before the drug is given. If positive, then drug desensitization may be indicated.
  ○ **Graded dose challenge:** This is performed by an allergy specialist in the presence of resuscitative equipment to minimize risk.
  ○ **Pretreatment protocols:** Medications causing anaphylactoid reactions may undergo premedication to reduce the incidence and severity of a reaction when the drug is administered.
  ○ **Perform desensitization:** Used when a type I hypersensitivity reaction is known, or when suspected, but no testing is available to evaluate. The procedure is performed by a trained allergist in an area with resuscitation equipment needed for anaphylaxis.

DIAGNOSIS

Clinical Presentation

• A thorough history is essential for making the diagnosis of an allergic drug reaction.
• Questions should be directed at establishing the following information:
  ○ Sign and symptoms: Where and what order did the symptoms begin, progress, and resolve?

○ Timing of the reaction: From the first dose of suspected drug, to the peak of the reaction, and resolution after discontinuing therapy.

○ Purpose of drug: Was it prescribed for the appropriate treatment and can the signs and symptoms be explained by a concurrent illness?

○ Other medications the patient is receiving: This includes all over-the-counter drugs and dietary supplements.

○ Prior exposure to the drug or another drug in the same or related class: If so, when was it given and what was the outcome?

○ History of other allergic drug reactions: Did the patient ever see an allergist and receive skin testing? What was the reaction and how long ago was the reaction?

• **Anaphylaxis** is discussed in detail in Chapter 13. It is important to remember that **anaphylactoid reactions** are indistinguishable from anaphylaxis, but it is not an IgE-mediated reaction.

• **Urticaria and angioedema** are discussed in detail in Chapter 9. An example of a type I hypersensitivity and the second most frequent drug-induced skin eruption.

• Fixed drug reaction: **Skin lesions that recur in the same area on reexposure to a drug.**

○ Typically the lesion is round and well delineated. Starts as an area of edema, then becomes erythematous and darkens to a violaceous colored area. The lesion is raised and non-pruritic.

○ Begins 30 minutes to 8 hours after re-exposure to the drug.

○ After withdrawal of the drug, the lesion will resolve in 2–3 weeks leaving an area of desquamation and then hyperpigmentation.

○ Drugs commonly implicated in fixed drug reactions include phenolphthalein, barbiturates, sulfonamides, tetracycline, and nonsteroidal antiinflammatory drugs (NSAIDs).

• **Serum sickness:** A type III hypersensitivity reaction with soluble immune complexes that activate the complement system.

○ Symptoms begin 6–21 days after administration of the drug and include fever, malaise, skin eruptions (palpable purpura or urticaria), arthralgias/myalgias, arthritis, lymphadenopathy, and leukopenia.

○ Once the offending drug is discontinued, symptoms resolve completely in a few days to weeks depending on the severity.

○ β-lactams are the most commonly associated nonserum drug to cause serum sickness.

• **Drug fever:** May be the only manifestation of a drug allergy. Fever may reach high temperatures.

○ Associated findings are leukocytosis, mild eosinophilia, elevated erythrocyte sedimentation rate (ESR), transaminitis, and rash.

○ After withdrawal of drug, defervescence occurs with 48–72 hours. If the drug is re-administered, fever recurs within hours. **Diagnosis is one of exclusion.**

• **Maculopapular or morbilliform skin eruptions:** The most common drug-induced skin eruption.

○ Rash typically is symmetric beginning in areas of pressure and spares the palms and soles.

○ It is confluent with erythematous macules and papules. Begins 4–7 days after initiating a drug.

• **Contact dermatitis:** Discussed in further detail in Chapter 11, is a type IV hypersensitivity reaction from exposure of a topically applied drug.

- **Erythema multiforme:** A skin eruption that is generally self-limited. Presents with a combination of macules, papules, vesicles, bullae, and targetoid lesions.
  - **Lesions are predominately on the extremities and involve the palms and soles**, but rarely the scalp or face.
  - **Mucosal involvement is usually limited to the oral cavity.** Rash resolves in 2–4 weeks and may have residual hyperpigmentation.
- **Erythema multiforme major** (Stevens–Johnson syndrome, SJS): A more severe manifestation, characterized by fever, mucosal involvement, and sloughing of <10% of the epidermis. Ocular involvement is common.
  - Symptoms begin 1–3 weeks after starting the drug. Recovery can last 6 weeks. Mortality around 10% in severe cases.
  - Discontinuing the offending drug and starting high dose corticosteroids reduce morbidity and mortality.[11]
  - **If the putative drug is re-administered, symptoms will recur and thus any drug challenge (including graded challenge) is contraindicated.**
  - Drugs that commonly cause SJS include sulfonamides, anticonvulsants, barbiturates, phenylbutazone, piroxicam, allopurinol, and aminopenicillins.
- **Toxic epidermal necrolysis** (TEN): TEN is life-threatening and characterized by **fever, diffuse necrosis, and sloughing of >30% of epithelial surface.**
  - TEN has a mortality rate of up to 40%.[12] There may be a benefit to treat TEN with intravenous immunoglobulin (IVIG).[13]
  - As with SJS, **any drug challenge (including graded challenge) with the offending agent is contraindicated.**
  - Drugs associated with TEN include sulfonamides, allopurinol, barbiturates, carbamazepine, phenytoin, and NSAIDs.
- **DIL:** Symptoms may not appear for months after initiating a drug. Patient may experience fever, malaise, arthralgias, and pleurisy.
  - Unlike idiopathic systemic lupus erythematosus (SLE), it is rare to have a butterfly malar rash, discoid lesions, oral ulcers, Raynaud phenomenon, alopecia, and renal or neurologic involvement.
  - DIL is seen in older individuals with males and females equally affected. It is a milder disease than SLE.
  - **Patients have a positive ANA or antihistone antibody.**
  - Symptoms resolve days to weeks after the drug is removed. Although, symptoms may persist for months before disappearing.
  - Drugs with the highest risk of DIL are hydralazine, procainamide, and quinidine.
- **Drug-induced hepatitis:** Begins 1–5 weeks after initiating drug. Liver damage may result from cholestasis, hepatocellular injury, or a mixture of both.
  - Patient may develop icterus, fever, rash, and eosinophilia in addition to abnormalities in the liver function tests.
  - Recovery can be expected after removal of the offending drug, if irreversible cell damage has not occurred.
  - Commonly offending agents include halothane, phenytoin, nitrofurantoin, allopurinol, phenothiazines, and sulfonamides.
- **Acute interstitial nephritis** (AIN): Symptoms start days to weeks after initiating the drug. Associated with fever, rash, and eosinophilia.
  - Renal involvement includes mild proteinuria, microhematuria, and eosinophiluria.
  - Renal insufficiency resolves once offending drug is removed.

○ Drugs seen in AIN are β-lactams (especially methicillin), rifampin, NSAIDs, sulfonamides, captopril, allopurinol, methyldopa, anticonvulsants, cimetidine, ciprofloxacin, and proton pump inhibitors.
- **Hematologic manifestations:** Usually appear without any other symptoms, onset is quick, and resolve in 1–2 weeks after discontinuing the drug. Drug-induced cytopenias are often due to type II hypersensitivity. Commonly implicated drugs for the following cytopenias are listed:
  ○ **Eosinophilia** can be caused by: gold salts, allopurinol, aminosalicylic acid, ampicillin, tricyclic antidepressants, capreomycin sulfate, carbamazepine, digitalis, phenytoin, sulfonamides, vancomycin, and streptomycin.
  ○ **Thrombocytopenia:** gold salts, quinidine, sulfonamides, and heparin.
  ○ **Hemolytic anemia:** PCN, cisplatin, tetracycline, methyldopa, levodopa, mefenamic acid, procainamide, tolmetin, quinidine, chlorpropamide, nitrofurantoin, probenecid, rifampin, streptomycin, isoniazid, erythromycin, ibuprofen, triamterene, and phenacetin.
  ○ **Neutropenia:** sulfonamides, sulfasalazine, propylthiouracil, semisynthetic PCNs, quinidine, procainamide, phenytoin, phenothiazines, cephalosporins, and gold.

Diagnostic Criteria

Table 14-1 presents the clinical criteria for an allergic drug reaction.[4]

TABLE 14-1 CLINICAL CRITERIA OF ALLERGIC DRUG REACTIONS
1. Allergic reactions occur in only a small percentage of patients receiving the drug and cannot be predicted from animal studies.
2. The observed clinical manifestations do not resemble known pharmacologic actions of the drug.
3. In the absence of prior exposure to the drug, allergic symptoms rarely appear before 1 week of continuous treatment. After sensitization, even years previously, the reaction may develop rapidly on reexposure to the drug. As a rule, drugs used with impunity for several months or longer are rarely the culprits. This temporal relationship is often the most vital information in determining which of many drugs being taken needs to be considered most seriously as the cause of a suspected drug hypersensitivity reaction.
4. The reaction may resemble other established allergic reactions, such as anaphylaxis, urticaria, asthma, and serum sickness-like reactions. However, various skin rashes (particularly exanthems), fever, pulmonary infiltrates with eosinophilia, hepatitis, AIN, and lupus syndrome have been attributed to drug hypersensitivity.
5. The reaction may be reproduced by small doses of the suspected drug or other agents possessing similar or cross-reacting chemical structures.
6. Eosinophilia may be suggestive if present.
7. Rarely, drug-specific antibodies or T lymphocytes have been identified that react with the suspected drug or relevant drug metabolite.
8. As with adverse drug reactions in general, the reaction usually subsides within several days after discontinuation of the drug.

Reprinted from: Ditto AM. Drug allergy: introduction, epidemiology, classification of adverse reactions, immunochemical basis, risk factors, evaluation of patients with suspected drug allergy, patient management considerations. In: Grammer LC, Greenberger PA, eds. *Patterson's Allergic Diseases*, 7th ed. Philadelphia, PA: Lippincott Williams & Wilkins, 2009:238–275, with permission.

Diagnostic Testing

- Diagnostic tests for allergy are discussed in further detail in Chapter 8.
- *In vivo* testing involves skin testing and test dosing the patient with the suspected drug.
  - **Prick and intradermal cutaneous tests** help to measure an IgE response. A patient with a positive wheal-and-flare response identifies a drug that can cause anaphylaxis.
    - HMW drugs such as antisera, egg-containing vaccines, monoclonal antibodies, latex, and toxoids can be used directly as skin testing reagents.
    - It is important for patients to abstain from using antihistamines and tricyclic antidepressants, which can interfere with the wheal-and-flare response.
    - There is a refractory period of 2–4 weeks after an episode of acute anaphylaxis where skin tests are invalid.
    - **A negative wheal-and-flare test does not rule out a drug allergy.**
  - **Patch testing** can be used to asses for a type IV contact hypersensitivity to topical agents.
    - A series of antigens are placed on the skin under occlusive dressing and results read 48–72 hours later.
  - **Graded dose challenge** (or provocative test dosing) provides a direct challenge to the patient to determine whether a suspected drug caused the clinical manifestations.
    - Graded challenges are generally performed when there is low probability of a true drug allergy.
    - However, this approach has the risk of a potentially serious adverse reaction and must be performed by a person with experience in managing hypersensitivity reactions.
    - In graded challenges, the dose of medication is incrementally raised until therapeutic dose is achieved.
    - This approach minimizes the risk of an adverse reaction by exposing the patient to progressively larger doses of the medication.
    - **If a patient tolerates a graded challenge without any adverse reaction, the patient does not have an allergy to the medication.** Future doses of the same medication can be administered without further testing.
    - Oral administration of provocative test dosing has a lower risk of serious adverse reaction than parenteral routes. **When possible, oral dose challenges are preferred over parenteral dose challenges.**
    - If the risk of an adverse reaction is felt to be too high to risk a graded challenge, a drug desensitization can be performed.
    - Graded dose challenges are faster than desensitizations but carry a higher risk of adverse reaction.
- *In vitro* testing uses various laboratory tests to aid in the assessment of drug allergy.
  - β-**tryptase levels** are elevated up to 8 hours after an anaphylactic event. It is more sensitive than serum or urine histamine levels.
  - Decreases in total hemolytic complement (CH50) or C3 and C4 levels can be seen in drug reactions involving complement activation.
  - Total IgE levels are not useful for drug allergy.
  - *In vitro* measurement of **antigen-specific IgE** can be helpful in diagnosing drug allergy.
    - In general, measuring *in vitro* antigen-specific IgE is less sensitive than skin testing.

- It requires the knowledge of which drug metabolite is immunogenic which is not known for many drugs.
- *In vitro* antigen-specific IgE has been validated for the major (penicilloyl) determinant of PCN, but not for the minor determinant.
- **The lack of an *in vitro* antigen-specific IgE to a drug does not rule out drug allergy.**

TREATMENT

- **Withdrawing the suspected culprit drug is the most important step in managing an ADR.**
- For the drugs that are essential, switching to another non–cross-reacting alternative agent is indicated.
- Most ADRs due to allergy will resolve with discontinuation of the offending agent.
- Follow practice guidelines for treatment of anaphylaxis (Chap. 13), urticaria, angioedema (Chap. 9), bronchospasm, and contact dermatitis (Chap. 11).
- Serum sickness reactions can be treated with antihistamines and NSAIDs. Prednisone taper can be given for severe reactions.
- SJS, drug fever, and DIL can be treated with corticosteroids.
- In TEN, corticosteroids are not effective but IVIG may play a role.
- Table 14-2 shows a commonly used **premedication protocol for RCM.**
- **Desensitization** can help prevent reactions. This procedure is performed only by a trained allergist in an area with resuscitation equipment needed for anaphylaxis.
  ○ The drug is given in 15–10 minute intervals in half-log10 increments until therapeutic dose is achieved.
  ○ Table 14-3 provides a sample desensitization protocol.[14]
  ○ The mechanisms underlying desensitization are not fully understood but **a successful desensitization will result in temporary tolerance to the medication.**
  ○ Patients will be tolerant to the medication only as long as the drug continues to be given. In general, **if the patient goes longer than 24 hours without a dose, then desensitization will need to be performed again.**
  ○ β-blockers should be withheld or tapered before procedure. Mild skin reactions such as urticaria or pruritus may occur and can be treated without discontinuing the procedure.
  ○ The choice to perform a graded dose challenge or desensitization should be based on the assessment of an experienced clinician.

TABLE 14-2	PRETREATMENT PROTOCOL FOR RADIOCONTRAST MEDIA		
Time before the procedure (hour)	Drug and dose		
	Prednisone[a]	Cimetidine[b]	Diphenhydramine[c]
13	50 mg PO or IV	300 mg PO or IV	
7	50 mg PO or IV	300 mg PO or IV	
1	50 mg PO or IV	300 mg PO or IV	50 mg PO or IV

[a]Or methylprednisolone, 40 mg IV.
[b]Or ranitidine, 150 mg.
[c]Or chlorpheniramine, 10–12 mg.

Time (minute)	Units	Route
0	100	PO
15	200	PO
30	400	PO
45	800	PO
60	1,600	PO
75	3,200	PO
90	6,400	PO
105	12,500	PO
120	25,000	PO
135	50,000	PO
150	100,000	PO
165	200,000	PO
180	400,000	PO
195	50,000	SC
210	100,000	SC
225	200,000	SC
240	400,000	SC
255	800,000	SC
270	1,000,000	IM
285	100,000	IV
300	200,000	IV
315	400,000	IV

TABLE 14-3 PROTOCOL FOR ORAL PENICILLIN DESENSITIZATION

Adapted from: Sullivan TJ, Wedner HJ. Drug allergy. In: *Allergy Theory and Practice*, 2nd ed. Philadelphia, PA: WB Saunders, 1992:548.

SPECIAL CONSIDERATIONS

Penicillin Allergy

- PCN allergy is the **most common cause of drug-induced anaphylaxis.**
- Anaphylaxis has been reported to occur in 1:100,000 with serious allergic reactions in 4.6 per 10,000 administrations.[15]
- As many as 10% of hospitalized patients report a history of allergy to PCN with many reporting a rash as the allergic reaction.
- PCN reactions can be stratified by time course (Table 14-4). Immediate (<1 hour) and accelerated reactions (1–72 hours) are IgE mediated.
- The most frequently reported PCN allergy is a maculopapular rash, which occurs in 2–3% of a treatment course. The next most common reactions include urticaria, fever, and bronchospasm.
- PCN requires conjugation with proteins to elicit an immune response given its LMW.
- **The major antigenic determinant is a penicilloyl moiety** formed by PCN covalently binding to lysine residues in serum or cell surface proteins. This occurs in approximately 93% of PCN molecules.

TABLE 14-4	PENICILLIN REACTIONS BY TIME COURSE	
Immediate (<1 hour)	**Accelerated (1–72 hours)**	**Delayed (>72 hours)**
Anaphylaxis	Urticaria	Maculopapular rash
Urticaria	Bronchospasm	Fever
Angioedema	Erythema multiforme	Serum sickness
Bronchospasm	Maculopapular rash	Recurrent myalgias or urticaria
	Serum sickness	

- The minor antigenic determinants are all remaining PCN conjugates (7%), which include penicillin, penicilloate, and penilloate.
- Skin testing:
  - The major antigenic determinant can be tested with Pre-Pen. It was withdrawn from the market in 2004 due to lack of a manufacturer, but has been FDA approved again in 2009. **Pre-Pen is the only FDA-approved skin test for drug allergy.**
  - A standardized test for minor antigenic determinants is not commercially available. A fresh solution of benzylpenicillin can be used for skin testing.
  - Skin testing will not help to predict the occurrence of a non–IgE-mediated reaction.
  - The predictive value of a history of PCN allergy and combination of skin testing in determining PCN hypersensitivity shows that 19% of patients with a positive history will have a positive skin test. In patients with a negative history of PCN allergy, 4–7% had a positive skin test. The incidence of reaction among skin test-negative subjects is <1% when evaluating for minor antigenic determinants.[16,17]
- Cross-reactivity:
  - The cross-reactivity between β-lactam antibiotics is variable and largely determined by their side-chain structure attached to the β-lactam nucleus.
  - **Cephalosporins** had higher cross-reactivity to PCN before 1980 as cephalosporins were contaminated with small amounts of PCN.[18] Risk of a cross-reaction with a first-generation cephalosporin is 5–16.5%, second generation is 4% and third or fourth generation 1–3%.[19]
  - Patients with **amoxicillin allergy** should avoid cefadroxil, cefprozil, and cefatrizine as all these drugs share same R-group side chain.
  - **Carbapenems** have been known to have increased cross-reactivity with PCN. Recent studies have shown that patients with a positive PCN skin test and negative carbapenem skin test underwent a graded carbapenem challenge, which did not result in any hypersensitivity reactions.[18]
  - The monobactam **aztreonam** rarely cross-reacts with PCN. Aztreonam does share an identical side chain as ceftazidime and are highly cross-reactive.[20]
- **Desensitization:** If there is no suitable alternative drug available and the patient has a positive skin test, then desensitization has to be performed. Table 14-3 shows a sample PCN protocol.

Sulfonamide Allergy

- Allergies to sulfonamides are increased in patients with HIV compared to the general population. TMP-SMX hypersensitivity occurs in 5% of HIV-negative patients and in 60% of patients with HIV.[9]

- The most common reaction is a **maculopapular rash** that develops 7–12 days after initiating the drug. This may be associated with a fever. Urticaria can be seen, but anaphylaxis is rare. SJS and TEN are known to be caused by sulfonamides.
- Sulfonamide antibiotics have a p-aminobenzoic acid ring that is similar to thiazides, furosemide, and sulfonylureas. Sulfonamides are metabolized primarily by N-acetylation and secondarily by cytochrome P450 N-oxidation.
- **Slow acetylators are at increased risk of drug reaction** as they preferentially metabolize sulfonamide antibiotics by N-oxidation resulting in reactive nitroso metabolites which cause cellular damage and react with protein to become immunogenic. This switch in metabolism is due to decreased glutathione reductase, which is also known to be diminished in HIV patients.[21]
- There are no standardized skin tests to evaluate sulfonamide drug allergy.
- Slow and rapid **desensitization** protocols have been established for sulfonamide allergy. A rapid protocol sample is listed in Table 14-5.[22]

Local Anesthetics

- Patients often report ADRs to local anesthetics (LAs), but these **rarely represent a true allergy.** The patient may have experienced a side effect of the epinephrine given with the LA or a vasovagal reaction.

TABLE 14-5	ORAL SULFONAMIDE DESENSITIZATION PROTOCOL (RAPID)	
Steps	**Concentration[a] (mg/mL)**	**Volume (mL)**
Phase I: Time interval between dosages is 15 minutes		
1–4	0.000008/0.00004	0.5; 1; 2; 4
5–8	0.00008/0.0004	0.5; 1; 2; 4
9–12	0.0008/0.004	0.5; 1; 2; 4
13–16	0.008/0.04	0.5; 1; 2; 4
17–20	0.08/0.4	0.5; 1; 2; 4
21–24	0.8/4	0.5; 1; 2; 4
25	8/40	0.5
Phase II: Time interval 30 minutes between doses		
1	8/40	1
2	8/40	2
Phase III: Time interval between doses		
1–4	8/40	2
5	8/40	3
6	8/40	5
7	8/40	8
8	8/40	10
9	80/400	1 tablet
10	80/400	Maintain with 1 tablet bid

[a]All dilutions are made from stock solution of trimethoprim 40 mg + sulfamethoxazole 200 mg/ 5 mL.

Adapted from: Kalanadhabhatta V, Muppidi D, Sahni H, et al. Successful oral desensitization to trimethoprim-sulfamethoxazole in acquired immune deficiency syndrome. *Ann Allergy Asthma Immunol* 1996;77:394–400.

TABLE 14-6	CLASSES OF LOCAL ANESTHETICS
PABA-containing	**Non–PABA-containing**
Chloroprocaine (Nesacaine)	Bupivacaine (Marcaine)
Procaine (Novocain)	Etidocaine (Duranest)
Tetracaine (Pontocaine)	Lidocaine (Xylocaine)
	Mepivacaine (Carbocaine)
	Prilocaine (Citanest)

PABA, p-aminobenzoic acid.

- LAs are divided into two classes based on the structure. Table 14-6 lists LAs.
  - p-aminobenzoic acid (PABA)-containing LAs (esters) cross-react with one another.
  - Non–PABA-containing LAs (amides) do not cross-react with one another or with PABA-containing LAs.
- The reliability of skin test for LAs has not been defined.
- If the LA causing the previous reaction is known, then choose another LA that does not cross-react.
- If the LA is unknown and the patient is to undergo a procedure, then contact the practitioner to test the LA of choice. Multiple LAs can be tested at once, such as one PABA-containing LA and two non–PABA-containing LA.
- Testing consists of **epicutaneous skin testing** using full-strength drug with positive and negative controls then followed by intradermal testing with 0.02 mL of drug diluted 1:100. If the skin testing is negative, then testing proceeds with subcutaneous incremental challenge using 0.1 mL of full-strength drug and graduating to 1 mL.[23]
- **It is important not to use a preparation containing epinephrine or preservatives for skin testing.** Epinephrine may cause false-negative skin test and parabens may cause false-positive skin test. Patients with a previous reaction should use preservative-free preparations in the future.
- If the reported allergic reaction was delayed in onset, then wait 24–48 hours to confirm a negative skin test before proceeding to challenge. Then wait another 24–48 hours after incremental challenge before using LA clinically.

REFERENCES

1. Johansson SG, Bieber T, Dahl R, et al. Revised nomenclature for allergy for global use: report of the nomenclature review committee of the World Allergy Organization, October 2003. *J Allergy Clin Immunol* 2004;113:832–836.
2. Lazarou J, Pomeranz BH, Corey PN. Incidence of adverse drug reactions in hospitalized patients: a meta-analysis of prospective studies. *JAMA* 1998;279:1200–1205.
3. Gomes ER, Demoly P. Epidemiology of hypersensitivity drug reactions. *Curr Opin Allergy Clin Immunol* 2005;5:309–316.
4. Ditto AM. Drug allergy: introduction, epidemiology, classification of adverse reactions, immunochemical basis, risk factors, evaluation of patients with suspected drug allergy, patient management considerations. In: Grammer LC, Greenberger PA, eds. *Patterson's Allergic Diseases*, 7th ed. Philadelphia, PA: Lippincott Williams & Wilkins, 2009:238–275.

5. Pichler WJ, Adam J, Daubner B, et al. Drug hypersensitivity reactions: pathomechanism and clinical symptoms. *Med Clin North Am* 2010;94:645–664.

6. Adkinson NF. Risk factors for drug allergy. *J Allergy Clin Immunol* 1984;74(4):567–572.

7. Enright T, Chua-Lim A, Duda E, et al. The role of a documented allergic profile as a risk factor for radiographic contrast media reaction. *Ann Allergy* 1989;62(4):302–305.

8. Mallal S, Nolan D, Witt C, et al. Association between presence of HLA-B*5701, HLA-DR7, and HLA-DQ3 and hypersensitivity to HIV-1 reverse-transcriptase inhibitor abacavir. *Lancet* 2002;359(9308):727–732.

9. Phillips E, Mallal S. Drug hypersensitivity in HIV. *Curr Opin Allergy Clin Immunol* 2007;7(4):324–330.

10. Bierman CW, Pierson WE, Zeitz SJ, et al. Reactions associated with ampicillin therapy. *JAMA* 1972;220(8):1098–1100.

11. Tripathi A, Ditto AM, Grammer LC, et al. Corticosteroid therapy in an additional 13 cases of Stevens-Johnson syndrome: a total series of 67 cases. *Allergy Asthma Proc* 2000;21(2):101–105.

12. Roujeau JC, Kelly JP, Naldi L, et al. Medication use and the risk of Stevens-Johnson syndrome or toxic epidermal necrolysis. *N Engl J Med* 1995;333:1600–1607.

13. French LE, Trent JT, Kerdel FA. Use of intravenous immunoglobulin in toxic epidermal necrolysis and Stevens-Johnson syndrome: our current understanding. *Int Immunopharmacol* 2006;6(4):543–549.

14. Sullivan TJ, Wedner HJ. Drug allergy. In: Korenblat PK, Wedner JH, eds. *Allergy Theory and Practice,* 2nd ed. Philadelphia, PA: WB Saunders, 1992:548.

15. Johannes CB, Ziyadeh N, Seeger JD, et al. Incidence of allergic reactions associated with antibacterial use in a large, managed care organisation. *Drug Saf* 2007;30(8):705–713.

16. Green GR, Rosenblum AH, Sweet LC. Evaluation of penicillin hypersensitivity: value of clinical history and skin testing with penicilloyl-polylysine and penicillin G. *J Allergy Clin Immunol* 1977;60:339–345.

17. Sogn DD, Evans R, Shepherd GM, et al. Results of the National Institute of Allergy and Infectious Diseases Collaborative Clinical Trial to test the predictive value of skin testing with major and minor penicillin derivatives in hospitalized adults. *Arch Intern Med* 1992;152:1025–1032.

18. Khan DA, Solensky R. Drug allergy. *J Allergy Clin Immunol* 2010;125(2 suppl 2):S126–S137.

19. Greenberger PA. 8. Drug allergy. *J Allergy Clin Immunol* 2006;117(2 suppl Mini-Primer):S464–S470.

20. Frumin J, Gallagher JC. Allergic cross-sensitivity between penicillin, carbapenem, and monobactam antibiotics: what are the chances? *Ann Pharmacother* 2009;43(2):304–315.

21. Davis CM, Shearer WT. Diagnosis and management of HIV drug hypersensitivity. *J Allergy Clin Immunol* 2008;121:826–832.

22. Kalanadhabhatta V, Muppidi D, Sahni H, et al. Successful oral desensitization to trimethoprim-sulfamethoxazole in acquired immune deficiency syndrome. *Ann Allergy Asthma Immunol* 1996;77:394–400.

23. DeShazo RD, Nelson HS. An approach to the patient with a history of local anesthetic hypersensitivity: experience with 90 patients. *Allergy Clin Immunol* 1979;63:387–394.

Insect Allergy

K. Lindsey B. McMullan

GENERAL PRINCIPLES

- Insects cause several types of reactions in individuals in the United States. Most stings produce a transient local reaction. A smaller subset can develop serious or life-threatening reactions.[1]
- The majority of stings that are caused by insects in the Order *Hymenoptera*, which includes bees, yellow jackets (YJs), wasps, hornets, and ants.
- Evaluation of sting reactions must include type of insect, type of reaction, necessity for auto-injectable epinephrine prescription, and necessity for referral to an allergy and immunology specialist.

Definition

- *Hymenoptera* (Latin for membranous wings) are insects with two pairs of wings, antennae, and an ovipositor that is used to deliver the venom. Families of interest include *Apidae, Vespidae,* and *Formicidae.*
- Apidae include **honeybees** (HBs) and **bumblebees.**
  - Domestic HBs are usually found in commercial hives.
  - Wild HBs build their nests in buildings, tree hollows, or old logs. They are typically not aggressive if not around their nests.
  - Usually stings are occupational. When they sting, a barbed stinger with venom sac is usually left behind. Most other insects do not leave a stinger, however, it is possible, so a stinger is not pathognomonic of the HB.
  - **Africanized HBs** can be found in the Southwestern states including California, Arizona, New Mexico, Texas, and Nevada. They attack in swarms and are much more aggressive than the domestic HB. Secondary to their swarming nature, many stings may occur causing a toxic reaction.[1]
- *Vespidae* includes YJs, wasps, and hornets.
  - YJs live in the ground, wall tunnels, logs, or crevices. **They are aggressive and responsible for most reported reactions.** They do not require much provocation for stinging, particularly around food.
  - **Hornets** have large paper-mâché nests that are often found in shrubs or trees. They are aggressive and may chase once provoked.
  - **Wasps** have smaller hives in a honeycomb shape. These can be found under eaves, patio furniture, and also in shrubs.
  - All three of these insects are attracted to human foods and can be found at outdoor events or around garbage.[1]
- *Formicidae* include fire ants and harvester ants.
  - **Fire ants,** particularly those in the genus *Solenopsis,* are most commonly found in the Southeastern and south central states.
    - They are native to South America.

- *Solenopsis invicta* venom causes a sterile pustule which is pathognomonic for a fire ant bite.[2]
  - ○ *Formicidae* differ from other *Hymenoptera* in that they do not have wings and sting in a circular pattern that causes the pustule.

Classification

- **Local reactions** are either small or large and immediate or delayed.
  - ○ Typically the area is swollen, red, and painful.
  - ○ By definition, a local reaction must be contiguous with the site of the sting.
  - ○ Immediate reactions occur within <4 hours.
- **Large local reactions** are defined by a diameter >10 cm with symptoms peaking in 24–48 hours.[3]
  - ○ These reactions can last for 5–10 days and can be so large as to include an entire extremity.
  - ○ Cutaneous symptoms must be contiguous.
  - ○ These reactions may be accompanied by fever, fatigue, and malaise.
- **Cutaneous systemic reactions** are similar to large local reactions except they are noncontiguous (e.g., a sting to the foot with a separate reaction appearing on the hand in a noncontiguous fashion). Signs are confined to the dermis and may include urticaria and angioedema.
- **Systemic reactions** include both cutaneous systemic reactions and anaphylaxis.
  - ○ Multiple systems may be included: Cardiovascular (hypotension and tachycardia), respiratory (bronchospasm, laryngeal edema, tongue swelling, or throat swelling), neurologic (seizures), gastrointestinal (GI) (nausea, emesis, diarrhea, abdominal pain).
  - ○ Anaphylaxis generally requires two or more body systems to be involved (see Chapter 13).
  - ○ If bradycardia is present, a vasovagal reaction should be considered, though anaphylaxis can occasionally present with bradycardia.[4]

Epidemiology

- Systemic reactions in US adults have a prevalence of approximately 3%. About 40 deaths occur in the United States each year secondary to insect stings.[1]
- Large local reactions occur more frequently and worldwide have a prevalence of 2.4–10%.
  - ○ Beekeepers have a higher prevalence, up to 38%.
  - ○ Those who sustain a large local reaction have a 5–15% chance of a systemic reaction if stung by the same type of insect again.[3]
- Children ≤16 years old that have a cutaneous systemic reaction have about a 10% chance of developing a systemic reaction if re-stung. The following reaction is most likely to be cutaneous.[1]
- Of those stung, about 30% will later be positive to venom-specific skin testing or venom-specific serum IgE (sIgE) testing.[5]
- **YJ or HB** will be positive on either skin testing or sIgE in 10–20% of all adults.[5] Of those evaluated for YJ or HB reaction, 30–50% will have a positive skin test to both.[6]
- **Fire ants** sting up to half of those they come in contact with each year.[7]

Pathophysiology

- Reactions to insect bites are caused by different mechanisms.
  - ○ **Most immune-mediated reactions are IgE-mediated.**

○ Other immune reactions have also been reported including the following:
  ■ Serum-sickness–like responses.
  ■ Neuritis.
  ■ Encephalitis.
  ■ Glomerulonephritis.
  ■ Vasculitis.
○ When stung by multiple insects simultaneously, the venom may cause a **toxic reaction.**
  ■ These reactions **may appear clinically similar to anaphylaxis** and can cause death.
  ■ Multiple stings, particularly with Africanized HB or fire ants, can be incited by disturbing a hive or nest.[1]
○ Components of venom which produce a damaging effect, but do not necessarily induce IgE, include hyaluronidase, melittin, mast cell degranulating peptide, mastoparan-C, histamine, dopamine, norepinephrine, acetylcholine, and kinins.[3,5]
- **Venom allergens causing IgE reactions consist of proteins.**
  ○ The major protein in **HB** is Api-m-1.
  ○ The major protein in YJ, *Vespula vulgaris,* is Ves-v-5.
  ○ The fire ant protein Sol-i-3 is similar to Ves-v-5.[6]
- Fire ant venom (solenopsin) strongly inhibits myocardial contractility.
  ○ This is thought to be from the alkaloid portion of the venom (95%).
  ○ It has been postulated that heart failure after a large number of fire ant stings could be secondary to this property of solenopsin.
  ○ The 5% of the venom that is protein leads to IgE-mediated reactions.[7]
- Reactions to biting insects, such as mosquitoes, deerfly, and Triatoma (kissing bug and bed bug) typically cause **itching and not pain.**
  ○ Their allergens generally come from salivary proteins and not venoms.
  ○ Anaphylaxis has been implicated in the deerfly and Triatoma.
  ○ Large local reactions are more typical of a bad reaction to a mosquito.
- Vespids have significant cross-reactivity (YJ, hornet, wasp).
  ○ Different species in the same genera of ants will cross-react; however, they do not have much cross-reactivity across genera [e.g., different species of fire ant (*Solenopsis*) cross-react with each other but not with harvester ants (*Pogonomyrmex*)].
  ○ HBs have very limited cross-reactivity with bumblebees.[5]

Risk Factors

- Risk for systemic reaction is based on severity of previous reaction, type of insect allergy, and time since previous reaction.
  ○ **The more severe the reactions, the greater the chance a subsequent reaction will be severe.**
  ○ For an anaphylactic reaction, if the patient is re-stung in the next 9 years, risk of anaphylactic response is 60%. Without intervention, this risk decreases to 40% if it has been 10–20 years since the previous sting.
  ○ **HB allergy confers a greater risk of systemic reaction** compared to other hymenoptera.[5]
- Occupation and hobbies can put you at risk for stings.
  ○ Beekeepers have the highest risk.
  ○ Gardeners, campers, farmers, and horseback riders also are at increased risk.
  ○ Risk for a sting also increases if you are in an outdoor area where food is present.

- Risk of systemic reaction is increased by the following[4]:
  - Angiotensin converting enzyme (ACE) inhibitors.
  - Baseline tryptase levels >5 ng/L.
  - Male sex.
- Elevation of baseline tryptase is independent risk factor for severe anaphylaxis to sting.[8]
- There is higher risk of future anaphylaxis if a patient had a serum sickness reaction, toxic reaction, had multiple stings at once, or had a previous sting within a few weeks.

DIAGNOSIS

- History is very important in helping to distinguish the type of insect.
- Physical characteristics of the reaction help determine future risk and what, if any, diagnostic workup needs to be pursued.
- *Hymenoptera* allergy is confirmed through allergen-specific IgE testing.

Clinical Presentation

History
- A key element of history is attempting to find out **what insect** stung the patient.
  - Both the nature and location of the activity occurring at the time of sting are important.
  - Any characteristics the patient can use to describe the insect are helpful as well such as size, color, or whether a stinger was left in the skin.
  - If the patient is able to actually bring in the insect, then an accurate diagnosis can be made.
- It is also important to note whether or not the patient actually saw an insect, or if there is an insect bite on examination. This assists in differential diagnosis as 25% of the general population have sensitization to venom on random testing.[5]
- Other important elements of history include assessment of:
  - Time from sting to reaction (**latency**).
  - **Duration** of the reaction.
  - History of **previous stings** (and by what insects).
- A thorough history of the patient's activities, hobbies, and other medical problems will help tailor treatment.
- Medical comorbidities and current medications can be prognostic. For example, patients on β-blockers can have protracted anaphylaxis.

Physical Examination
- Physical examination should focus on type of reaction (local or systemic) and then further characterize (large local, cutaneous systemic, anaphylaxis).
- **Cardiovascular** collapse is responsible for 25% of fatalities. Important signs include flushing, tachycardia, hypotension, and vascular collapse/shock.
- **Respiratory** obstruction is responsible for 60% of fatalities. Important signs include lip, tongue, and/or throat angioedema, wheezing, stridor, and respiratory distress or failure.
- **Cutaneous** symptoms include pain and pruritus.
  - Signs include the distribution of swelling, contiguity of swelling, flushing, urticaria, and whether or not there is angioedema of lip, throat, or tongue.

- ○ Pustules present at the bite area are pathognomonic of fire ants.
- ○ Size of the swelling and contiguity are very important in determining whether the reaction is local, large local, or systemic.
- **GI** symptoms include nausea and abdominal cramping. Signs include emesis and diarrhea.
- **Other general signs and symptoms** to watch for are dizziness, fainting, seizures, malaise, fever, fatigue, rashes indicative of vasculitis, joint pain, renal, mental, or sensory complaints.
- Evaluation for signs of secondary **infection** at bite site(s). Septicemia is the cause of 2% of deaths.

Diagnostic Criteria

- Correct classification leads to appropriate diagnostic workup, treatment, and assessment of prognosis.
- **Large local** reactions are >10 cm with symptoms peaking in 24–48 hours. Swelling and erythema must be contiguous.
- **Cutaneous systemic** reactions have non-contiguous areas of swelling and erythema.
- **Systemic anaphylaxis** requires signs in two or more systems (e.g., swelling with erythema and hypotension).
- **To make a definitive diagnosis, venom-specific IgE testing by either skin prick or radioallergosorbent testing (RAST) must be performed and be positive in light of a convincing history.**[1]

Differential Diagnosis

- Other illnesses can be confused with an insect sting, particularly if the insect was not seen.
- Diagnoses to consider include the following:
  - ○ Local:
    - Cellulitis
    - Vasculitis
    - Boils
    - Abscess
  - ○ Systemic:
    - Vasovagal reaction
    - Myocardial infarction
    - Pulmonary embolism
    - Sepsis
    - Drug reaction
    - Food allergy
    - Other cause of anaphylaxis

Diagnostic Testing

- Diagnostic testing focuses primarily on identifying the culprit insect so that venom immunotherapy (VIT) may be instituted.
- If the diagnosis of anaphylaxis is in question, a **serum tryptase** can be drawn within 1–4 hours after the event and followed up after the patient is stabilized.
- **Testing should be performed to all members of** *Hymenoptera* **unless the patient can absolutely identify fire ant as the stinging insect.** If fire ant is identified, testing with venom to other stinging insects is not indicated.[1]

- Further diagnostic testing to identify type of insect is indicated in anaphylaxis, systemic cutaneous reaction, and some large local reactions.
- Diagnostic testing typically begins with immediate hypersensitivity testing with positive and negative controls. **It is preferable to wait 3–6 weeks after having a reaction before skin testing is performed to prevent false negatives.**
- Skin prick testing can be performed to a number of insects.
  - **In the United States testable venom proteins include yellow hornet, white faced hornet, YJ, wasp, and HB.**
  - Epicutaneous testing is followed by intradermal skin testing if the results are negative.
  - Testing is considered positive if a response occurs at or before 1.0 μg/mL of venom or 1:500 wt/vol for fire ant extract.
  - The size of a positive skin test does not necessarily correlate to the severity of the reaction.
- If skin testing is negative and the patient has had a systemic reaction, repeat skin testing should be performed at a return clinic visit, or *in vitro* venom-specific sIgE testing should be performed prior to deciding that VIT is not necessary.
- Venom-specific sIgE testing should be used in lieu of skin testing in patients with severe skin conditions or who are dermatographic. **Skin testing is preferable if possible as it is more sensitive.**

TREATMENT

Medications

Immediate Therapy for a Sting
- Local reactions are treated symptomatically.
  - Pain relief can be obtained with cold compresses and oral analgesics.
  - Oral antihistamines may help the itching.
- Patients with large local reactions can also be treated with **oral antihistamines and analgesics.**
- In addition, **oral steroids** (40–60 mg tapered over 0–5 days) can be prescribed if edema is spreading, limbs are not functioning properly, or edema involves the lip or face.[3,5]
- **For anaphylaxis, epinephrine is the treatment of choice.**
  - **In a life-threatening situation, there is no contraindication for epinephrine.**[1]
  - If anaphylaxis occurs, the patient should be monitored for at least 3–6 hours for a late-phase reaction or protracted anaphylaxis, particularly if they are taking β-blockers.
  - Glucagon may be helpful for patients on β-blockers.[5]
- **Auto-injectable epinephrine** is available by prescription at doses of 0.3 mg administered IM or 0.15 mg administered IM. Individuals weighing more than 30 kg should receive 0.3 mg dosing.
- Individuals who are prescribed auto-injectable epinephrine should be educated on how to use these devices properly.

Venom Immunotherapy
- Table 15-1 summarizes who should receive VIT.
- VIT is indicated in patients who have had a systemic reaction, anaphylaxis, and in some patients who have experienced large local reactions. Patients must have demonstration of venom-specific IgE either by skin or *in vitro* testing.

TABLE 15-1	GENERAL GUIDELINES FOR VENOM IMMUNOTHERAPY
Reaction	**Is venom immunotherapy indicated?**
Local reaction (small)	No
Large local reaction	Based on individual circumstance, usually No
Anaphylaxis	
Mild/dermal in children	No
Mild/dermal in adults	Yes
Moderate or severe	Yes
Serum sickness	Yes

- VIT is a potentially lifesaving treatment for patients with systemic reactions to *Hymenoptera.*
- VIT decreases the risk of future systemic reaction to less than 5%.[1]
- VIT is generally recommended for those older than 16 who have experienced cutaneous systemic reaction.
- Exceptions do exist if the parent desires VIT or if the patient is at high risk for frequent or multiple stings.[1]
- Patients who have large local reactions and work in an occupation or participate in hobbies with high risk of multiple or frequent stings should be considered for VIT.[6]
- VIT is composed of the venoms (or whole body extract in the case of fire ant) to which a given patient is allergic.
  - Components of VIT are determined by antigen-specific IgE testing.
  - All venoms a patient tests positive to are generally used.
- VIT requires a commitment by the patient.
  - Injections are generally administered once weekly until a few weeks after the maintenance dose is reached (100 μg venom or 0.5 mL of 1:100 wt/vol fire ant extract) after which dosing is spaced to 4-week intervals.
  - It can take up to 28 weeks to reach maintenance assuming there is no reaction to the treatments.
  - VIT should be continued for 3–5 years.
  - The decision of when to discontinue VIT is still being debated and should be a decision between the patient and the physician based on numerous factors such as type of insect, future risk of stings, and type of reaction to insect sting.[1,9]
- Reactions to VIT can be local or systemic.
  - The majority are local, though 5–15% can have systemic reactions.
  - Systemic reactions are more likely in those treated with HB and in patients with underlying mast cell disease.
  - Pretreatment with oral antihistamines may help to reduce all reactions.[5]
- Secondary to the risk of severe reactions, VIT should be administered in a medical office capable of treating anaphylaxis.
- If a patient takes a β-blocker and an alternative medication is not an option, extreme caution should be used when proceeding with VIT due to the risk of decreased response to therapy for allergic reactions.[1]

Lifestyle/Risk Modification

- Day-to-day preventive measures include the following:
  - ○ Have a professional exterminate nests in the area.
  - ○ Watch for new nests.
  - ○ Avoid bright or floral clothing when outside.
  - ○ Do not walk bare-foot outside.
  - ○ If working outside, wear clothing that covers skin including gloves, long pants/sleeves, head covering, socks with shoes.
  - ○ Exercise caution in high-risk areas such as attics, bushes, or picnics.
  - ○ Keep insecticides for use if a stinging insect is identified.
- Those with a history of systemic reaction or anaphylaxis should:
  - ○ Wear a medical alert necklace or bracelet.
  - ○ Carry auto-injectable epinephrine.
    - It should be reinforced that this medication should be **easily available**, and if sting occurs, its use should **not be delayed.**
    - Antihistamines are not a suitable substitute for epinephrine.
- It is prudent to discuss an emergency plan and remind patients to go to an emergency facility for monitoring if a sting occurs.
- For those who might be candidates for VIT it is important to refer them to an allergist-immunologist for venom-specific IgE testing.[1]

SPECIAL CONSIDERATIONS

- Pregnant patients can still receive VIT if it has already been started prior to pregnancy.
  - ○ VIT should not be initiated during pregnancy secondary to risk of effect of systemic reactions on the fetus.
  - ○ Dose should be maintained and not escalated in those pregnant women who are already on VIT.
  - ○ The patient and physician should weigh the small risk systemic reaction to VIT against risk of anaphylaxis to insect sting.
- Elderly patients are at higher risk for severe anaphylaxis.[6]
- The indications for VIT in children 16 years of age and younger differ from adults.

REFERRAL

See Table 15-2 for indications for referral.

TABLE 15-2	INDICATIONS FOR REFERRAL TO ALLERGIST-IMMUNOLOGIST

Patients who have:
Systemic reaction to a sting (cutaneous or anaphylactic)
Anaphylaxis with insect sting in the differential of causative factors
A reaction that may require venom immunotherapy
A comorbidity making anaphylaxis difficult to treat (e.g., on β blocker)
A need for further education on avoidance and treatment
A specific request to see an allergist–immunologist

MONITORING/FOLLOW-UP

- Initial monitoring after a systemic reaction should be at least 3–6 hours. Further care required can then be determined.
- Patients with systemic reactions should be referred to an allergist–immunologist for venom-specific IgE testing.
- For those undergoing VIT, they will receive an injection weekly until maintenance is achieved, and then be able to space out their injections.

OUTCOME/PROGNOSIS

- The majority of deaths occur **within 4 hours** of the sting, though 10% are delayed.
- For those who are undergoing a systemic reaction, the greatest factor determining prognosis will be use of epinephrine.
- Prognosis is good for those undergoing VIT. It decreases the risk of a systemic reaction to less than 5%.
- For those who have had a systemic reaction and do not receive VIT, risk for further systemic reaction can approach 60%.[1]
- The severity of future reactions is predicted by the severity of past reactions.
- 5–10% of those with large local reactions will have a systemic reaction in the future.[6]

REFERENCES

1. Moffitt JE, Golden DB, Reisman RE, et al. Stinging insect hypersensitivity: a practice parameter update. *J Allergy Clin Immunol.* 2004;114:869–886.
2. Hoffman DR. Ant venoms. *Curr Opin Allergy Clin Immunol.* 2010;10:342–346.
3. Severino M, Bonadonna P, Passalacqua G. Large local reactions from stinging insects: from epidemiology to management. *Curr Opin Allergy Clin Immunol.* 2009;9:334–337.
4. Demain JG, Minaei AA, Tracy JM. Anaphylaxis and insect allergy. *Curr Opin Allergy Clin Immunol.* 2010;10:318–322.
5. Golden DBK. Insect allergy. In: Adkinson NF, Busse WW, Holgate ST, et al., eds. *Middleton's Allergy: Principles and Practice,* 7th ed. Philadelphia, PA: Mosby/Elsevier, 2009:1005–1018.
6. Hamilton RG. Diagnosis and treatment of allergy to hymenoptera venoms. *Curr Opin Allergy Clin Immunol.* 2010;10:323–329.
7. deShazo RD. My journey to the ants. *Trans Am Clin Climatol Assoc.* 2009;120:85–95.
8. Rueff F, Przybilla B, Bilo MB, et al. Predictors of severe systemic anaphylactic reactions in patients with Hymenoptera venom allergy: importance of baseline serum tryptase-a study of the European Academy of Allergology and Clinical Immunology Interest Group on Insect Venom Hypersensitivity. *J Allergy Clin Immunol.* 2009;124:1047–1054.
9. Golden DB. Discontinuing venom immunotherapy. *Curr Opin Allergy Clin Immunol.* 2001; 1:353–356.

Food Allergy and Other Adverse Food Reactions

Amanda Trott

GENERAL PRINCIPLES

Definition

- **Adverse food reaction:** Any abnormal reaction due to ingestion of a food. This includes immunologic (allergy) as well as nonimmunologic reactions (food intolerances, e.g., lactose intolerance).[1]
- **Food allergy (FA):** Also referred to as food hypersensitivity, is an adverse health effect arising from a specific immunologic response that occurs reproducibly on exposure to a given food. This includes both immunoglobulin E (IgE)-mediated and non–IgE-mediated immunologic reactivity to specific foods.
  - ○ **IgE-mediated FAs** are FAs mediated by IgE. This requires both the presence of food antigen-specific IgE and the development of specific signs and symptoms upon exposure to a specific food.
  - ○ **Non–IgE-mediated FAs** are conditions that are immunologically mediated processes with reproducible signs and symptoms on exposure to a food but without IgE sensitization.

Classification

- The various forms of FA are presented in Table 16-1.
- **Food intolerances** are non–immune-mediated adverse reactions to food. Intolerance may result from metabolic, toxic, pharmacologic, or other causes.
- **Food-induced anaphylaxis** is an IgE-mediated, rapid-onset, serious systemic reaction which may result in shock and/or respiratory compromise.
- **Gastrointestinal (GI) food allergies:**
  - ○ **Immediate GI hypersensitivity:** IgE-mediated FA with upper GI symptoms within minutes (most commonly vomiting) and lower GI symptoms that are either immediate or delayed up to several hours.
  - ○ **Eosinophilic esophagitis (EoE):** Localized eosinophilic inflammation of the esophagus involving both IgE- and non–IgE-mediated mechanisms. Symptoms include vomiting, reflux, abdominal pain, dysphagia, and food impaction. Food avoidance frequently results in resolution.
  - ○ **Eosinophilic gastroenteritis:** Like EoE, but involving portions of the GI tract distal to the esophagus.
  - ○ **Dietary protein–induced proctitis/proctocolitis:** Presents in infants who seem healthy but have visible blood in the stool. This process is generally non–IgE-mediated, and differentiated from other GI food allergies with similar stool findings by lack of systemic symptoms. There is no specific testing, so the causal role of food allergens is inferred from a characteristic history on exposure.

TABLE 16-1 FOOD ALLERGIES

Disease	Subtype	Symptoms	Epidemiology	Diagnostic tests
IgE-mediated food allergy	Anaphylaxis	Hypotension, shock	All ages	SPT, *in vitro* antigen-specific IgE, OFC
	Cutaneous	Minutes to 2 hours: urticaria, angioedema, flushing, acute morbilliform rash, acute contact urticaria	All ages	SPT, *in vitro* antigen-specific IgE, OFC
	Respiratory	Acute rhinoconjunctivitis, acute bronchospasm	All ages	SPT, *in vitro* antigen-specific IgE, OFC
	Acute gastrointestinal hypersensitivity	Minutes to 2 hours: nausea, emesis, diarrhea, typically with cutaneous and/or respiratory symptoms	All ages	SPT, *in vitro* antigen-specific IgE, OFC
	Oral allergy syndrome	Pruritus, tingling, erythema or angioedema of the lips, tongue, oropharynx; immediately on contact of raw fruit with oral mucosa	All ages, most common in birch pollen-allergic young adults	SPT or OFC with raw fruits or vegetables
IgE- and cell-mediated food allergy	Allergic eosinophilic esophagitis	Chronic/intermittent GE reflux, emesis, dysphagia, abdominal pain, food impaction	All ages, but especially infants, children, adolescents	50% have positive SPT and/or food-IgE; endoscopy and biopsy for conclusive diagnosis
	Allergic eosinophilic gastroenteritis	Chronic/intermittent abdominal pain, emesis, poor appetite, failure to thrive, weight loss, anemia, protein-loss	All ages	50% have positive SPT and/or food-IgE; endoscopy and biopsy for conclusive diagnosis
	Asthma	Chronic cough, wheezing, dyspnea	All ages, food allergy is a risk factor for intubation in children with asthma	SPT, *in vitro* antigen-specific IgE, OFC

Non-IgE-mediated food allergy	Atopic dermatitis	Relapsing pruritic vesiculopapular rash	Infants and children; 60–80% significantly improve/resolve by adolescence	SPT, *in vitro* antigen-specific IgE, OFC, elimination diet
	Allergic proctocolitis	Blood-streaked or occult blood positive stools, otherwise healthy-appearing	Infants <6 months, often breast-fed; usually outgrown by age 1	Resolution of blood loss in 48 hours after allergen elimination
	Food protein–induced enterocolitis syndrome	Subacute repetitive emesis, dehydration, diarrhea	Young infants, breast-feeding is protective; usually outgrown by age 1–3 years	Response to dietary restriction, OFC
	Dietary protein–induced enteropathy	Protracted diarrhea, emesis, failure to thrive, often anemia	Young infants; usually outgrown by age 1–2 years	
	Celiac disease	Chronic diarrhea, malabsorption, abdominal distention, flatulence, failure to thrive or weight loss, possibly oral ulcers and/or dermatitis herpetiformis	All ages	Endoscopy and biopsy, response to dietary restriction
				Biopsy diagnostic; screen with serum IgA antitissue transglutaminase and antigliadin; resolution with gluten elimination
	Contact dermatitis	Relapsing pruritic eczematous rash, often to hands or face; occupational food contact	All ages, more common in adults	Patch testing

IgE, immunoglobulin E; SPT, skin prick test; OFC, oral food challenge; GE, gastroesophageal.

○ **Food protein–induced enterocolitis syndrome (FPIES):** Non–IgE-mediated disorder presenting in infants with very severe vomiting and diarrhea, most commonly caused by cow's milk, soy, or grains.

○ **Oral allergy syndrome (OAS):** Localized IgE-mediated allergy to fresh fruits or vegetables, with itching, tingling, and/or swelling of the lips, tongue, roof of the mouth, and throat. This affects patients with pollen allergy and is also referred to as pollen-associated FA syndrome.

• **Cutaneous reactions to foods:**

○ **Acute urticaria:** A common manifestation of IgE-mediated FA, especially in the setting of anaphylaxis, with rapid development of polymorphic, round, or irregularly shaped pruritic wheals after ingestion of the problem food.

○ **Angioedema:** Typically IgE-mediated when food-induced and usually in combination with urticaria. This is a nonpitting, nonpruritic, well-defined swelling of the subcutaneous tissues, abdominal organs, or upper airway. Also a common feature of anaphylaxis.

○ **Atopic dermatitis (AD):** Because this disease involves complex interaction between skin barrier dysfunction and environmental factors, the role of FA in its pathogenesis remains controversial. In some sensitized patients, food allergens can aggravate AD.

○ **Acute contact dermatitis:** A form of AD caused by cell-mediated allergic reactions to chemical haptens in foods, resulting in pruritus, erythema, papules, vesicles, and edema.

○ **Contact urticaria:** Can be either immunologic (IgE-mediated) or non-immunologic (direct histamine release).

• **Respiratory manifestations:** These are important components of anaphylaxis but are uncommon in isolation.

Epidemiology

• **Food allergies are over-reported by patients,** which is one of many obstacles in establishing the true prevalence of FA.

• Objective measurements are necessary to make an accurate FA diagnosis.

• **Milk, egg, and peanut account for the vast majority of allergic reactions in young children.**

• **Peanut, tree nuts, and seafood account for the vast majority of reactions in teenagers and adults.**

• The following data are drawn from a recent meta-analysis of 51 publications[2]:

○ Self-reported FA to cow's milk, hen's eggs, peanuts, fish, or crustacean shellfish: 13% for adults, 12% for children.

○ When objective measures were employed, including skin test, serum IgE, or food challenge, the overall prevalence dropped to 3% for all ages.

• US prevalence rates for specific foods[1]:

○ Peanut allergy: 0.4–0.8%.

○ Tree nut allergy: 0.4%.

○ Seafood allergy: 0.6% in children, 2.8% in adults.

• **Most children with FA will eventually tolerate cow's milk, egg, wheat, and soy but far fewer eventually tolerate peanut and tree nuts.**

• **Allergy to seafood most commonly develops in adulthood and usually persists.**

• A high initial level of allergen-specific IgE to a food is associated with a lower resolution rate over time.

• The resolution of AD is a useful marker for the onset of tolerance to food allergens.

- A decrease in the level of allergen-specific IgE is often associated with the ability to tolerate foods.

Pathophysiology

- In the normal mature gut, about 2% of ingested food antigens penetrate the GI tract barrier and enter the circulation.[3]
- The majority of individuals develop what is known as **oral tolerance** to these antigens, which is a state of **immunologic unresponsiveness**.
- A failure to develop tolerance or a breakdown in this process results in excessive production of food-specific IgE antibodies.
- When food allergens penetrate the mucosal barriers and reach these antibodies bound to mast cells or basophils, mediators are released, which result symptoms of **immediate hypersensitivity**, including vasodilation, smooth muscle contraction, and mucus secretion (type I hypersensitivity).
- These cells also may release cytokines and other mediators that contribute to a late-phase response.
- The clinical manifestations of IgE-mediated hypersensitivity are widely variable but depend on various host and antigen factors.
- As for non–IgE-mediated food reactions, pathogenic factors are not well defined, but, like IgE-mediated FA, likely involve a break in oral tolerance resulting in an inappropriate immune response to orally ingested antigens.

Risk Factors

- Biologic parents or siblings with existing, or history of, allergic rhinitis, asthma, AD, or FA increase risk of FA.
- Presence of AD, especially when severe with early onset, is associated with increased risk of food sensitization.
- **Asthma is the risk factor most commonly identified with the greatest severity of allergic reactions to foods.**
- Complementary factors that affect the absorption of a food allergen may increase the severity of a reaction and should be taken into account. These include concomitant alcohol consumption, use of nonsteroidal anti-inflammatory drugs (NSAIDs), and exercise.

Prevention

The following are **not** recommended, as there is insufficient evidence to support the idea that such practices prevent the development or clinical course of FA:
- Limited exposure to non-food allergens (e.g., dust, pollen, pet dander) even for those patients considered to have increased risk for the development of FA.
- Routine FA testing prior to the introduction of allergenic foods.
- Maternal diet restriction during pregnancy or lactation.
- Use of soy infant formula instead of cow's milk infant formula in at-risk infants.
- Delayed introduction of solid foods beyond 4–6 months of age.

Associated Conditions

- Children with FA are 2.3 times more likely to have asthma, 2.3 times more likely to have AD, and 3.6 times more likely to have respiratory allergies than children without FA.[1]
- Asthmatics that also have FA are more likely to have increased rates of emergency department visits and hospitalization in an intensive care unit for their asthma than non-food allergic asthmatics.

- EoE is frequently associated with FA.
- Exercise-induced anaphylaxis in adults is triggered by foods about one-third of the time, according to patient report.

DIAGNOSIS

Clinical Presentation

- Manifestations of an immune-mediated reaction to food can vary widely.
- Most IgE-mediated reactions are considered to be immediate, meaning they occur within minutes to a few hours.
- Delayed responses occur within several hours to a few days and are thought to involve cellular mechanisms.
- **Food-induced anaphylaxis** (see Chap. 13) is the most common, serious consequence of FA.
  - ○ Typically IgE-mediated and believed to involve systemic mediator release from sensitized mast cells and basophils.
  - ○ Significantly under-recognized and under-treated.
  - ○ Prompt recognition and management is essential to ensure a favorable outcome.
  - ○ Fatalities can occur within 30 minutes of exposure and usually result from respiratory compromise.

Differential Diagnosis

- Acute allergic reactions triggered by other allergens, such as medications or insect stings.
- AD flares triggered by other irritants.
- Chronic GI symptoms due to reflux, infection, anatomical abnormalities, or metabolic disorders.
- Chemical and irritant effects of foods, such as gustatory rhinitis due to neurologic responses to temperature or capsaicin.
- Gustatory flushing syndrome is an erythematous band on the cheek in the distribution of the auriculotemporal nerve, triggered by tart foods.
- Food poisoning due to bacterial toxins or scombroid poisoning.
- For those with eosinophilic GI disorders, other diagnoses such as parasitic infections, GI reflux disease (GERD), systemic eosinophilic disorders, and vasculitis should be considered.
- Mental/behavioral disorders resulting in food aversion.
- Pharmacologic effects such as tryptamine in tomatoes and food additives may mimic allergic symptoms of the skin and GI tract.

Diagnostic Testing

- Diagnostic testing is based on a comprehensive history, which should suggest whether or not the reaction was IgE- or non–IgE-mediated. This determines the kind of testing to pursue and the possible foods involved.
- **Testing should not be comprised of general broad panels of food allergens.**

Laboratories
- **Total serum IgE:**
  - ○ Although it is often elevated in atopic individuals, it **not a sensitive and specific test for FAs.**

○ Obtaining this study for the purpose of providing a ratio of food-specific IgE to total IgE offers no advantage over food-specific IgE alone in the diagnosis of FA.
- **Food allergen-specific serum IgE:**
  ○ Formerly measured using the radioallergosorbent test (RAST), **specific IgE levels are now measured by more sensitive fluorescence enzyme-labeled assays.**
  ○ Similar to skin prick text (SPT) in the sense that these tests are useful in indentifying foods that may be provoking IgE-mediated food allergic reactions but are **not diagnostic of FA alone.**
  ○ Very useful in detecting allergic sensitization, meaning the presence of allergen-specific antibodies; sensitization does not always correlate with clinical allergy.
  ○ Especially useful when SPT cannot be done, either due to clinical contraindications or failure to discontinue antihistamines prior to the test.
  ○ Studies support the idea that specific IgE antibody levels directly correlate with likelihood of clinical reactivity.[4]
- **Mast cell and basophil mediators:**
  ○ Histamine and tryptase are rarely used to support the diagnosis of food-induced anaphylaxis.
  ○ **Tryptase lacks specificity and may not be elevated in food-induced anaphylaxis.**

Diagnostic Procedures

Skin Prick Test
- SPT assists in the identification of foods that potentially induce IgE-mediated reactions but is **not diagnostic of FA when used alone.**
- It reflects the IgE bound to cutaneous mast cells.
- SPT has a **low positive predictive value,** as many patients have IgE to certain foods without clinical FA.
- When the patient provides a history very suspicious for FA, SPTs are valuable in identifying the foods responsible, and therefore have **high sensitivity and a high negative predictive value** in this clinical setting.
- Results are immediately available, making SPT the most commonly performed procedure in the evaluation of IgE-mediated FA.
- The patient **must be off all antihistamine medications for 1 week** prior to the procedure to insure the reliability of the test.

Intradermal Tests
- This method is not more sensitive than SPT in detecting food protein–induced allergic reactions.
- The risk of systemic adverse allergic reactions is greater compared to SPT.
- Intradermal tests are **rarely indicated** for the evaluation of FA.

Other
- **Oral food challenges:**
  ○ **The double-blind placebo-controlled food challenge is the gold standard for diagnosing FA,** but its use is limited by time and expense.
  ○ Single-blind and open food challenges are frequently used to screen patients for FA.
  ○ Should be designed and performed under medical supervision and avoided in patients with a recent life-threatening reaction to a particular food.

- **Food elimination diets:**
  - Cutting out one or a few specific foods may be useful in the diagnosis of FA, especially in the setting of non–IgE-mediated disorders such as FPIES.
  - Prolonged elimination diets consisting of multiple foods are **not** recommended.

TREATMENT

Medications

Epinephrine
- Prompt and rapid IM epinephrine after onset of symptoms of anaphylaxis is **first-line therapy.**
- **Benefits of epinephrine far outweigh the risks** and delays in epinephrine administration are associated with increased morbidity and death.
- Dosing:
  - Autoinjector (IM): 0.15 mg for individuals 10–30 kg; 0.3 mg for those >30 kg.
  - Epinephrine IM 1:1,000 solution: 0.1 mg/kg, maximum dose of 0.3 mg.
- The anterior-lateral thigh is the preferred injection site.
- IV epinephrine is recommended for patients who do not respond to IM epinephrine and whose fluid status may not be adequate for muscle perfusion.
- **Repeated epinephrine dosing is required up to 20% of the time** and can be done every 5–15 minutes in patients with ongoing or progressive symptoms.
- After epinephrine administration, the patient should be transferred to an emergency facility for observation for at least 4–6 hours and possible further treatment.

Adjunctive Treatment
- Epinephrine is the only first-line treatment for anaphylaxis, and there is no substitute.
- The following treatments are adjunctive, and there are little or no data demonstrating their effectiveness:
  - Inhaled β2-agonist every 20 minutes or continuously as needed.
  - Antihistamines: Diphenhydramine 1–2 mg/kg/dose, maximum 50 mg IV or oral (preferably liquid for ready absorption); ranitidine 1–2 mg/kg/dose, max 150 mg oral and IV.
  - Prednisone 1 mg/kg oral or methylprednisolone 1 mg/kg IV, maximum 60–80 mg for both.
  - Oxygen therapy.
  - Large volume IV fluids.
  - Recumbent positioning with lower extremities elevated.
  - In the hospital setting, vasopressors or glucagon can be given for refractory hypotension.

Discharge Therapy
- Epinephrine autoinjector prescription/instructions, allergen avoidance education, follow-up with primary care physician, consider referral to an allergist.
- Adjunctive over the next 48–72 hours: Diphenhydramine every 6 hours, ranitidine twice daily, and prednisone.
- There are no medications that are currently recommended for the prevention of IgE- or non–IgE-mediated food allergic reactions.

Milder Food Allergic Reactions
- Symptoms such as flushing, urticaria, mild angioedema, or OAS can be treated with antihistamines.
- If progression is noted, epinephrine should be given immediately.
- If the patient has a history of prior severe allergic reaction, epinephrine should be given earlier in the course.

Immunotherapy for Food Allergy
While allergen-specific immunotherapy has been shown to improve clinical symptoms of FA for some patients, it is **not recommended at this time because of the risk of severe reaction combined with unclear long-term efficacy in preventing future food-allergic reactions.**

Lifestyle/Risk Modification
Diet
- **Allergen avoidance is currently the safest strategy for managing IgE-mediated and non–IgE-mediated FA.**
- Food allergen avoidance in patients with documented FA may reduce the severity of associated comorbid conditions such as AD and EoE.

SPECIAL CONSIDERATIONS

Vaccinations in Patients with Egg Allergy
- Many vaccines are grown in chick embryos and may contain small, variable amounts of egg protein.
- The MMR (measles, mumps, and rubella) and MMRV (measles, mumps, rubella, and varicella) vaccines are safe in egg-allergic children, even in those with a history of severe reaction to egg.
- Influenza:
  - Either the inactivated or live-attenuated vaccine should **not** be given to children with history of:
    - Egg-allergic symptoms with co-existent asthma or
    - Systemic anaphylaxis to egg.
  - Unless:
    - The vaccine contains <1.2 µg/mL of ovalbumin or
    - The patient has had a negative result on skin prick testing with the vaccine.
  - In the case of positive SPT, the vaccine can be given but the dose should be divided: One-tenth followed by the remainder if the initial dose is tolerated.
- Rabies and yellow fever vaccines should **not** be given to patients with egg allergy, unless an allergy evaluation and testing to the vaccine has been done.

PATIENT EDUCATION

Food Labeling
- Patients with FAs and their caregivers must be educated on the interpretation of ingredient lists on food labels to optimize trigger avoidance.
- In 2004, a law was passed by the US Congress requiring that **products containing any of the eight major food allergens must clearly list them on the label in simple English.** This includes peanut, tree nuts, egg, milk, soy, wheat, fish, and shellfish.

Emergency Management

- Patients with FAs and their caregivers should be informed on the risk of anaphylaxis and should be able to recognize signs and symptoms early.
- Families should be equipped with the knowledge and skills to handle such medical emergencies, including understanding of and ready access to an anaphylaxis emergency action plan.
- Epinephrine autoinjector teaching should be done in the office and the clinician should ensure that the patients/caregivers are familiar with the sequence of events according to the action plan.
- Patients should wear medical identification jewelry or carry an anaphylaxis wallet card.

MONITORING/FOLLOW-UP

- Annual testing is reasonable to evaluate whether a patient has outgrown allergy to those foods that are likely to resolve over time (e.g., milk, egg, wheat, and soy), assuming the patient has not had a recent reaction to those foods.
- Testing for ongoing allergy to peanut, tree nuts, fish, and shellfish should not be performed more frequently than every 2 to 3 years since allergy to these foods is not typically outgrown quickly.

REFERENCES

1. NIAID-Sponsored Expert Panel, Boyce JA, Assa'ad A, Burks AW, et al. Guidelines for the diagnosis and management of food allergy in the United States: report of the NIAID-sponsored expert panel. *J Allergy Clin Immunol.* 2010;126:S1–S58.
2. Rona RJ, Keil T, Summers C, et al. The prevalence of food allergy: a meta-analysis. *J Allergy Clin Immunol.* 2007;120:638–646.
3. Sampson HA, Burks AW. Adverse reactions to foods. In: Adkinson N, et al., eds. *Middleton's Allergy: Principles and Practice,* 7th ed. Philadelphia, PA: Elsevier, 2009:1139–1163.
4. Sampson HA. Utility of food-specific IgE concentrations in predicting symptomatic food allergy. *J Allergy Clin Immun.* 2001;107:891–896.

Latex Hypersensitivity

17

Eric Karlin

GENERAL PRINCIPLES

Definition

- **Latex hypersensitivity** refers to immunologic reactions, both immunoglobulin E (IgE)-mediated and cell-mediated, when sensitized individuals are exposed to latex-containing materials.[1]
- **Latex allergy (LA)**, however, refers only to immediate hypersensitivity reactions caused by exposure to products containing natural rubber latex in persons with latex-specific IgE. Clinical reactions include **urticaria, asthma, rhinoconjunctivitis, or even anaphylaxis.**
- **Latex sensitivity** is diagnosed in patients with elevated levels of latex-specific IgE or a positive latex skin test. It **does not necessarily indicate clinical allergy** but rather the presence of a latex-specific IgE.

Epidemiology

- Although there was a dramatic increase in reported LA with the institution of universal precautions in the 1980s, more recent years have seen a decrease in the incidence of LA, likely due to improvements in the manufacturing process and creation of latex-safe environments.
- A recent meta-analysis has estimated the prevalence of latex *sensitivity* to be between 0.5% and 5% for the general population and between 2.5% and 13% for health care workers.[2]
- It is estimated that **LA occurs in 4–5% of the health care worker population, which is three times more prevalent LA than in the general population.**[2]
- Increased prevalence of LA has been reported among patients with spina bifida and those with a history of multiple surgeries early in life.[3]

Pathophysiology

- Natural rubber is a highly processed plant product derived from the milky sap of the rubber tree *Hevea brasiliensis.*
- The harvested rubber is then processed in one of two ways:
  - Most latex is coagulated by acid to create molded rubber products such as catheters and pneumatic tires for vehicles.
  - Alternatively, latex may be ammoniated with the addition of accelerators, antioxidants, and preservatives to create dipped latex products.
- Dipped latex products are used to create latex gloves and are thought to carry the highest allergen content and cause most anaphylactic reactions to natural rubber latex.
- There are currently 13 known *Hevea* latex allergens, Hev b 1 through Hev b 13, that have been identified using molecular techniques.[1] Hev b 1 and Hev b 3 are major

allergens for children with multiple congenital anomalies, whereas Hev b 2, Hev b 4, and Hev b 5 are involved in LA among health care workers.[1]
- 30–50% of patients who are natural rubber latex allergic show an associated allergy to some foods, especially kiwi, banana, avocado, peach, tomato, potato, and bell pepper. This association, known as the **latex-fruit syndrome,** is due to cross-reactivity of epitopes between phylogenetically similar plant proteins.[4] Proteins involved include chitinase, β-1,3-glucanase, profilin, and lipid transfer protein.[4]

Risk Factors

Risk factors for the development of latex hypersensitivity include atopy, health care workers, non–health care workers with occupational exposure to latex, and children with spina bifida or genitourinary abnormalities who have undergone multiple surgeries.

DIAGNOSIS

Clinical Presentation

- **Irritant contact dermatitis** is the most common reaction to latex products and is often confused with latex hypersensitivity.
  - It is a **non-immunologic reaction** causing erythema, scaling, and fissures on the dorsum of the hand.
  - This condition is secondary to the irritant effects of repeated hand washing, occlusion from sweat, and an alkaline glove pH.
- **Allergic contact dermatitis** (see also Chap. 11) refers to a delayed-type hypersensitivity that occurs 1 or 2 days after contact with latex.
  - Patients present with erythema, pruritus, and vesicles with crusting on the dorsum of the hands.
  - This response is a **cell-mediated type IV hypersensitivity reaction** to additive oxidants and accelerator chemicals that are used in the latex manufacturing process rather than Hev b antigens.[5]
- **Allergic contact urticaria is an IgE-mediated immediate-type hypersensitivity to natural rubber proteins** and is the most common allergic reaction reported by health care workers who use latex gloves.[6] Patients present with **urticarial lesions 10–15 minutes after gloves are worn.**
- **Rhinoconjunctivitis and asthma** may occur when sensitized patients inhale latex allergens adsorbed by cornstarch powder found in gloves. This type I immediate hypersensitivity may induce ocular itching, tearing, rhinitis, and wheezing.
- **Anaphylaxis** has been reported when sensitive individuals are exposed to latex products.
  - Although anaphylaxis is rare, most episodes occur during surgical procedures, childbirth, gynecologic examinations, or dental procedures.[7]
  - Anaphylaxis has also been associated with inhalational exposure.

Diagnostic Testing

- **Skin testing** with natural rubber latex is widely performed in Europe and Canada to identify those individuals sensitive to latex products.
  - Currently, **no commercial skin test reagent is available in the United States.**[8]
  - Allergists in the United States have attempted skin testing by creating their own reagents in the office using *Hevea* latex products. Unfortunately, these products

vary widely in their allergen contents and systemic reactions have been reported with the use of these non-standardized preparations.

○ Nevertheless, skin prick tests with latex extracts may be considered in patients with a strong clinical history and negative serologic testing.[9]

- **Serologic testing** for the detection of latex-specific IgE may be performed when clinically indicated. **None of the assays can demonstrate complete diagnostic reliability** and results must be interpreted in the context of the clinical suspicion for LA.
- **Provocational challenge studies** have been performed on patients with negative results from serologic or skin prick testing when they have strong clinical histories that support LA.
  ○ Various tests including closely monitored glove use, nasal provocation, and inhalation challenge have been performed.[6]
  ○ The usefulness of these tests is limited by the widely varying allergen contents of latex gloves from different manufacturers. For this reason, many of these procedures are typically limited to research procedures and are not used clinically.
- **Patch testing** using a standard screening panel containing the additive oxidant and accelerator chemicals that are used in the latex manufacturing process may be used to help distinguish irritant contact dermatitis from allergic contact dermatitis.[10]

TREATMENT

- The mainstay of latex hypersensitivity and LA management focuses on **avoidance of latex products.**
- All latex-sensitive individuals should be educated on all personal and medical products that may contain latex.
- Because most IgE-mediated reactions to latex occur in health care workers or latex-sensitive individuals undergoing medical procedures, efforts have been placed to create "latex-safe" clinics and hospitals.
  ○ Prior to hospital admission and surgical procedures, screening questions should be asked to identify patients with possible latex sensitization (Table 17-1).
  ○ Once LA is detected, documentation and education regarding latex avoidance is imperative.
  ○ Establishment of a "latex-safe" environment through creation of a latex committee and establishment of an institutional program has been widely successful in decreasing latex-induced symptoms.[11]

TABLE 17-1	SCREENING QUESTIONS FOR LATEX SENSITIZATION

Have you ever had any past skin reaction, nasal or ocular allergic reaction, difficulty breathing, cough or wheezing, or anaphylactic shock reaction after contact with gloves, condoms, balloons, or other latex-containing products, or after a medical or dental procedure?

Do you have a personal or family history of atopy (allergies, hives, eczema, or asthma)?

Do you have a history of multiple surgeries or catheterizations?

Have you had any past allergic reaction to avocado, banana, chestnut, kiwi, potato, or tomato?

TABLE 17-2	LATEX-CONTAINING PRODUCTS
Medical	**Household**
Gloves	Toys
Catheters (including urinary catheters and wound drains)	Balloons
	Elastic on clothing
Tape	Mouse pads
Electrode pads	Condoms
Rubber syringe stoppers	Shoes
Tourniquets	Erasers
Face masks	Sporting goods
Ambu bags	Rubber handles on tools
Mattresses	Buttons on stereos, video cassette recorders, televisions, and remote controls
Patient-controlled analgesia syringes	
Stethoscope and BP cuff tubing	

- ○ It is recommended that all latex-containing products be removed from all hospital environments of any patient with LA, and that a latex-free operating room should be constructed for these patients.
- The FDA has established guidelines for labeling of any medical devices containing latex. A brief list of medical and household products that may contain latex is given in Table 17-2.
  - ○ Alternatives to latex gloves include vinyl, nitrile, neoprene, and styrene gloves.
  - ○ **Vinyl** gloves are similar in cost to latex gloves but are less protective against viral penetration.
  - ○ **Neoprene and styrene** gloves are used mostly for surgical purposes and are five to ten times more expensive that latex gloves.
  - ○ **Nitrile** gloves appear to be most comparable to latex gloves; however, they are produced with the same accelerator used in the production of latex gloves and may cause irritant or contact dermatitis.
- **Immunotherapy** for the treatment of IgE-mediated LA has been studied using both subcutaneous immunotherapy and sublingual immunotherapy. However, results have varied, and a high frequency of adverse events was reported in multiple studies.[12,13]
- Further information on lists of latex products and latex-free substitutes may be found through the Spina Bifida Association of America (http://www.sbaa.org) and the American Latex Allergy Association (http://www.latexallergyresources.org).

REFERENCES

1. Poley GE, Slater JE. Latex allergy. *J Allergy Clin Immunol.* 2000;105:1054–1062.
2. Bousquet J, Flahault A, Vandenplas O, et al. Natural rubber latex allergy among health care workers: a systematic review of the evidence. *J Allergy Clin Immunol.* 2006;118:447–454.
3. Niggemann B. IgE-mediated latex allergy: an exciting and instructive piece of allergy history. *Pediatr Allergy Immunol.* 2010;21:997–1001.
4. Wagner S, Breiteneder H. The latex-fruit syndrome. *Biochem Soc Trans.* 2002;30:935–940.
5. Pecquet C. Allergic contact dermatitis to rubber: clinical aspects and main allergens. *Clin Rev Allergy.* 1993;11:413–419.

6. Kurtz KM, Hamilton RG, Adkinson NF. Role and application of provocation in the diagnosis of occupational latex allergy. *Ann Allergy Asthma Immunol.* 1999;83:634–639.

7. Yunginger JW. Latex-associated anaphylaxis. *Immunol Allergy Clin N Am.* 2001;21:669–677.

8. Hamilton RG, Adkinson NF. Natural rubber latex skin testing reagent: safety and diagnostic accuracy of non-ammoniated latex, ammoniated latex and latex rubber glove extracts. *J Allergy Clin Immunol.* 1996;98:872–883.

9. Lieberman P, Nicklas RA, Oppenheimer J, et al. The diagnosis and management of anaphylaxis practice parameter: 2010 update. *J Allergy Clin Immunol.* 2010;126:477–480.

10. Neuget AI, Ghatak AT, Miller RL. Anaphylaxis in the United States: an investigation into its epidemiology. *Arch Intern Med.* 2001;161:15–21.

11. Bernstien DI, Karnani R, Biagini RE, et al. Clinical and occupational outcomes in health care workers with natural rubber latex allergy. *Ann Allergy Asthma Immunol.* 2003;90:209–213.

12. Leynadier F, Herman D, Vervloet D, et al. Specific immunotherapy with a standardized latex extract versus placebo in allergic healthcare workers. *J Allergy Clin Immunol.* 2000; 106:585–590.

13. Sastre J, Quirce S. Immunotherapy: an option in the management of occupational asthma? *Curr Opin Allergy Clin Immunol.* 2006;6:96–110.

Conditions Associated with Eosinophilia

18

Bob Geng

GENERAL PRINCIPLES

Definition

- **Eosinophilia** is defined as peripheral blood eosinophil count $>0.5 \times 10^9$ cells/L.
- The term **hypereosinophilia** applies to $>1.5 \times 10^9$ cells/L eosinophil count in the peripheral blood.[1]

Classification

- **Allergic diseases:** Atopic disease (allergic rhinitis, allergic asthma) and drug-induced.
- **Infectious diseases:** Parasitic (helminthes) and fungal (*Aspergillus* spp. [allergic bronchopulmonary aspergillosis (ABPA)] or coccidioidomycosis).
- **Hematologic and neoplastic:** Hypereosinophilic syndrome (HES), leukemia, lymphoma, tumor-associated mastocytosis.
- **Diseases with specific organ involvement:** Skin, pulmonary, gastrointestinal (GI) disorders, and renal disorders.
- **Immunologic reactions:** Immunodeficiency and transplant rejection.
- **Endocrine disorders:** Hypoadrenalism.
- **Miscellaneous disorders:** Atheroembolic disease and serosal irritation.

Pathophysiology

- Eosinophils are bone marrow–derived granulocytes involved in allergic and nonallergic inflammation.
- Average survival in the peripheral circulation ranges from 6–12 hours but in tissue survival time increases to several weeks.
- Eosinophils contain and can release large amounts of **preformed cytotoxic basic proteins** from intracellular granules. They include major basic protein, eosinophil cationic protein, eosinophil peroxidase, and eosinophil-derived neurotoxin.
- Eosinophils can also produce **superoxide, leukotrienes, and various inflammatory cytokines.**
- These cytotoxic proteins are involved in the host **defense against parasites.** However, when released near host cells, they can cause significant damage by promoting inflammation, thrombosis, angiogenesis, and connective tissue formation.
- Eosinophil growth factor cytokines include interleukin (IL)-5, IL-3, and granulocyte macrophage colony-stimulating factor (GM-CSF); the elevation of these cytokines lead to eosinophilopoiesis and prolongation of eosinophil survival time via inhibition of eosinophil apoptosis.
- Diurnal variations of peripheral blood eosinophil count occurs with the peak at night and trough in the morning—inversely proportional to the circulating endogenous adrenocorticosteroid level.[2]

- Peripheral blood eosinophil count is not always indicative of the degree of eosinophil activity because they are **primarily tissue-dwelling cells.** There can be several hundred times more eosinophils in particular tissues than in the blood.[2]
- The presence of increased amount of eosinophils in tissue usually denotes a pathologic condition.
- The arbitrary threshold of 1.5×10^9 cells/L has been classically used as the peripheral blood level to suggest possibility of sufficient tissue infiltration of eosinophils to cause target-organ damage. However, there is no precise correlation between peripheral blood level and target organ infiltration.[1]
- **Allergic disease is the most common etiology of eosinophilia in North America,** but parasitic infection is the most common etiology globally.
- Allergic disease and drug reactions are usually only associated with mild eosinophilia ($<1.5 \times 10^9$ cells/L); if the level of eosinophilia is above that, it raises the possibility of more serious underlying conditions.
- Specific mechanisms of disease processes will be discussed separately under differential diagnosis.

DIAGNOSIS

Clinical Presentation

History

- Medication history is very important since it may lead to the discovery of a temporal relationship between the initiation of a **new medication** with the onset of eosinophilia due to drug reaction.
- **Travel history:** Since many eosinophilic disorders can be caused by **parasitic infections,** it is essential to determine whether the patient has traveled to any tropical environments or developing countries particularly those that are endemic to certain parasitic infections commonly associated with eosinophilia. The temporal relationship of the travel and the onset of eosinophilia need to be determined.
- **Social history:** Need to determine possible **occupational or home allergen exposures.**
- Review of systems: Since eosinophilic conditions can affect many organ systems and can manifest in a myriad of syndromes, it is crucial to take a detailed review of systems in order to assess for presence of constitutional symptoms as well as any target-organ involvement or damage.

Differential Diagnosis

Allergic Diseases

- Allergic rhinitis is associated with nasal tissue eosinophilia.
- Both nasal and blood eosinophilia can be associated with the nonallergic rhinitis with eosinophilia syndrome (NARES).
- Chronic sinusitis is associated with both tissue and blood eosinophilia.
- Both allergic and nonallergic asthma is associated with airway tissue eosinophilia and allergic asthma is associated with blood eosinophilia.
- Careful environmental and allergen history may reveal pertinent exposures.

Medication-Induced Causes

- Careful medication history is necessary for evaluation, especially any new drugs.
- Eosinophilia can occur independent of systemic manifestations or organ dysfunction.

- **Interstitial nephritis:**
  - Common offending agents include penicillin, nonsteroidal antiinflammatory drugs (NSAIDs), cimetidine, sulfonamides, captopril, allopurinol, diphenylhydantoin, rifampin, ciprofloxacin, aztreonam, triazolam, and warfarin.
  - Eosinophiluria in acute interstitial nephritis is only 40–60% sensitive.[3]
- **Hepatitis:** Minocycline, choline magnesium trisalicylate, halothane, methoxyflurane, salicylazosulfapyridine, ranitidine, carbamazepine, phenytoin, and sulfa antibiotics.
- **Pulmonary eosinophilia:** Many antimicrobial agents, NSAIDs, dantrolene (both pleural and blood eosinophilia).
- **Drug rash, eosinophilia, and systemic symptoms (DRESS):**
  - DRESS can occur weeks after starting several types of medications including aromatic anticonvulsants (i.e., phenytoin, carbamazepine, and phenobarbital), dapsone, minocycline, sulfonamides, allopurinol, and nevirapine.[1,4]
  - Common signs include lymphadenopathy, high-grade fever, and organ involvement. Skin lesions are diffuse, progressively evolving, and pruritic.
- **Eosinophilia-myalgia syndrome** is a systemic adverse reaction to ingestion of substances containing L-tryptophan; pulmonary involvement was noted in 50–60% of cases.
- **Toxic oil syndrome** is associated with ingestion of oil contaminated with denatured rapeseed oil.
- **Cytokine therapies:** High doses of GM-CSF and IL-2 can lead to eosinophilic myocarditis and biventricular thrombosis.[5]

Infectious Causes
- **Helminthic infections:**
  - Eosinophilia may be a clue to the presence of helminthic infection.
  - Helminths that are sequestered within tissues or contained in the intestinal lumen may not present with blood eosinophilia.
  - Occasional leakage of fluids from echinococcal cysts may lead to transient increases in blood eosinophilia causing allergic response and/or anaphylactic reactions.
  - In the United States, *Strongyloides, Ascaris, Toxocara,* and *Ancylostoma* are the most common parasites causing pulmonary infiltrates.
  - *Strongyloides* infection can be indolent for decades causing eosinophilia. The use of corticosteroids for eosinophilia in patients with occult infection may lead to disseminated, possibly fatal, infection.
- Most **protozoan parasites** do not elicit blood eosinophilia except for *Dientamoeba fragilis* and *Isospora belli.*[2]
- **Fungal infections:** ABPA and coccidioidomycosis.
- **Retroviral infections:**
  - HIV with leucopenia leading to relative eosinophilia, medication-related, and adrenal insufficiency from opportunistic cytomegalovirus (CMV) infection.
  - HTLV-1 infections.

Hematologic and Neoplastic Disorders
- **Hypereosinophilic syndrome (HES):**
  - Persistent eosinophilia of >1,500 cells/μL.
  - No identifiable parasitic, allergic, or eosinophilic syndrome etiology.
  - Signs and symptoms of organ involvement.
  - HES affects men more than women at ratio of 9:1 and generally present from ages 20–50, but there are also pediatric cases.[6]

○ Common symptoms include fatigue, cough, dyspnea, myalgia, angioedema, rash, fever, and retinal disease.

○ Organ systems affected include cardiovascular, cutaneous, neurologic, pulmonary, GI, and hepatic.

○ **Cardiac involvement of HES:**

   ■ The pathogenesis involves stages.

   ■ First acute necrosis happens in the initial weeks of illness and presents with endocardial damage, myocardial infiltration with eosinophils and lymphocytes with formation of microabscesses. During this acute setting patients may develop subungual and/or conjunctival splinter hemorrhages.

   ■ Second, thrombus begins to form on the wall of the damaged endocardium.

   ■ Lastly, the fibrotic stage occurs with scarring leading to restrictive cardiomyopathy and entrapment of the chordae tendineae with consequent development of valvular disease.

○ **Neurologic involvement of HES:**

   ■ Embolic strokes and transient ischemic attacks (TIAs) from intracardiac thrombus formation can still occur even on warfarin and antiplatelet agents.[2]

   ■ Behavioral changes may include confusion, ataxia, and memory loss with upper motor neuron signs.

   ■ Peripheral neuropathy represents 50% of all neurologic manifestations.

• **Leukemia:**

   ○ Acute eosinophilic leukemia is a rare subtype of acute myeloid leukemia (AML).

   ○ Eosinophilia can also be a manifestation of the M4E0 subtype of AML.

   ○ Eosinophilia can be a feature of chronic myelogenous leukemia (CML) as well.

   ○ It is generally not seen in acute lymphoblastic leukemia (ALL).

• **Lymphoma:**

   ○ Peripheral blood eosinophilia can be seen in some patients with Hodgkin's and non-Hodgkin's lymphoma.

   ○ The involvement with Hodgkin's disease is generally attributed to the expression of IL-5 mRNA by Reed–Sternberg cells.

   ○ Certain B-cell lymphomas may be associated with eosinophilia.

   ○ Eosinophilia with eczema can be seen in cutaneous T-cell lymphoma.

• **Mastocytosis:**

   ○ Peripheral blood eosinophilia is seen in approximately 25% of systemic mastocytosis cases.[2]

   ○ See Chapter 19 for a more detailed discussion of mastocytosis.

• **Solid tumors:**

   ○ Large cell nonkeratinizing cervical tumors.

   ○ Large cell undifferentiated lung cancer.

   ○ Various mucosal membrane squamous cell carcinomas.

   ○ Adenocarcinoma of the GI tract and uterus as well as transitional cell carcinoma of the bladder can be associated with varying levels of eosinophilia.

Dermatologic Disorders

• Eosinophilia may be associated with **general dermatologic conditions** including atopic dermatitis, bullous pemphigoid, pemphigus vulgaris, psoriasis, dermatitis herpetiformis, herpes gestationis, and chronic urticaria.

• **Eosinophilic panniculitis:** Nodular lesions caused by infiltration of eosinophils into the subcutaneous fat. This condition is often associated with gnathostomiasis (also known as larva migrans profundus), leukocytoclastic vasculitis, and erythema nodosum.

- **Episodic angioedema with eosinophilia:** Presents with episodic angioedema with eosinophilia, urticaria, pruritus, fever, and weight gain. Serum IgM is often elevated. Excellent long-term prognosis and is usually steroid-responsive.[2]
- **Kimura's disease:** Large subcutaneous masses on the head and neck of Asian males associated with eosinophilia.
- **Angiolymphoid hyperplasia with eosinophilia:** Similar to Kimura's disease but with smaller superficial lesions and can occur in any race.
- **Eosinophilic fasciitis (Shulman's syndrome):** Acute presentation of swelling, erythema, and induration of the extremities often precipitated by exercise. Blood eosinophil level is elevated. The major pathology occurs in the subcutaneous tissues. MRI is the imaging study of choice for diagnosis and monitoring.
- **Eosinophilic cellulitis (Well's syndrome):** Recurrent episodes of cellulitis-like swelling of the extremities with minimal tenderness, no warmth, and not responsive to antibiotic therapy. Peripheral blood eosinophilia can be seen in half of the patients. The lesion generally resolves spontaneously.[2]
- **Eosinophilic ulcer of the oral mucosa:** Multiple ulcerated tender lesions affecting the tongue that is often precipitated by trauma. The lesions generally resolve spontaneously over a month.
- **Eosinophilic pustular folliculitis:** Seen in HIV or other immunosuppressed patients.
- **Recurrent cutaneous necrotizing eosinophilic vasculitis:** Eosinophilic infiltration of the lumen and vessel walls of small dermal vessels. Eosinophilic vasculitis can be associated with connective tissue disorders and hypocomplementemia. These patients generally respond to steroid treatment and have good prognosis.[2]

Pulmonary Disorders
- The pulmonary disorders associated with eosinophilia and their relationship to asthma are presented in Table 18-1.
- **Chronic eosinophilic pneumonia:**
  ○ Insidious onset (>1 month) of cough, fever, night sweats, dyspnea, weight loss. Less than one-third of patients have sputum production or wheezing.
  ○ Male to female ratio is 1:2 and the peak incidence is in fifth decade of life.[2]
  ○ Half of the patients have atopic disease and some patients have comorbid asthma.
- **Acute eosinophilic pneumonia (AEP):**
  ○ Acute onset between 1–5 days of cough, dyspnea, fever, pleuritic chest pain, hypoxemic respiratory failure, and myalgias.

TABLE 18-1	PULMONARY DISORDERS WITH EOSINOPHILIA
Associated with asthma	**Not associated with asthma**
ABPA	Bronchocentric granulomatosis
Chronic eosinophilic pneumonia	Chronic eosinophilic pneumonia
Churg–Strauss syndrome	Drug reaction
Tropical pulmonary eosinophilia	HES
	Löffler's syndrome
	Neoplasia
	PEG

ABPA, allergic bronchopulmonary aspergillosis; HES, hypereosinophilic syndrome; PEG, pulmonary eosinophilic granuloma.

○ Male predominant.

○ The exact etiology is unknown but AEP may be a form of acute hypersensitivity reaction to inhaled allergens.

○ AEP has been associated with NSAIDs, antidepressants, new-onset smoking, and parasitic infections.

- **Churg–Strauss syndrome:**
  ○ Characterized by hypereosinophilia, systemic vasculitis, and asthma.
  ○ Asthma and eosinophilia may precede vasculitis in many of patients.
  ○ Vasculitis of small- and medium-sized vessels.
  ○ Classical clinical presentation consists of an asthma patient with sinus disease, neuropathy, constitutional symptoms (fever, weight loss, and fatigue), and vasculitis that may affect the skin, heart, GI tract, kidney, or nervous system.
  ○ Cutaneous lesions include maculopapular erythematous rash, petechiae, purpura or ecchymoses, and tender nodular lesions.
  ○ Diagnostic criteria are four out of the six following features: Asthma, eosinophilia >10%, neuropathy, pulmonary infiltrates, sinus abnormalities, and tissue eosinophilia on lung biopsy.[7]

- **Löffler's syndrome (helminthic larval transpulmonary migration):**
  ○ The larva of *Ascaris,* hookworms, and *Strongyloides* transit through the blood, penetrate into the alveoli and migrate through the airway to enter the GI tract through the esophagus. The migration through the airway generally takes place 9–12 days after the ingestion of helminthic eggs. Ascaris is the most common parasite that causes Löffler's syndrome and is most likely to elicit symptoms.[2]
  ○ The typical clinical presentation (acute symptoms generally resolve between 5 and 10 days) includes nonproductive cough, burning substernal pain, rales, and wheezing.

- **Tropical pulmonary eosinophilia:**
  ○ This is an immune response to the microfilarial stages of *Wuchereria bancrofti* and *Brugia malayi* in the lung.
  ○ Endemic to Asia, Indian subcontinent, Africa, South America, and the Caribbean.
  ○ The clinical presentation may include constitutional symptoms (e.g., weight loss, fever, night sweats, and fatigue), dyspnea, and asthma symptoms (nocturnal cough and wheezing), and hemoptysis.

- **Drug- and toxin-induced eosinophilic lung disease:**
  ○ Many drugs are associated with pulmonary eosinophilia including methotrexate, nitrofurantoin, sulfa compounds, gold, salicylates, and antiepileptics.
  ○ Toxic occupational exposures include aluminum silicate, sulfite exposure in grape workers, and chemical fume exposure by rubber workers.[2]
  ○ The clinical presentation ranges from simple pulmonary eosinophilia to severe symptoms such as AEP.

- ABPA is discussed in Chapter 4.

- **Pulmonary eosinophilic granuloma (PEG):**
  ○ PEG is a rare fibro-inflammatory disease with interstitial infiltrates composed of eosinophils, lymphocytes, and Langerhans cells.
  ○ It is thought to be a type of Langerhans cell histiocytosis, derived from CD1+ and HLA-DR Langerhans cells.
  ○ Clinical presentation includes pleuritic chest pain, dyspnea, weight loss, fever, and hemoptysis.
  ○ Bone involvement may be associated with erosive lesions from expansion of cells in the medullary cavity. PEG should be suspected when patients develop insidious onset of cough in setting of these bony lesions.

- ○ PEG is also association with cigarette smoking.[2]
- ○ Spontaneous pneumothorax has been associated with PEG.
- ○ Eosinophils are found in lesions, but it is not usually associated with blood eosinophilia and not seen in the airways.
- ○ Spontaneous resolution has been seen but it may progress to pulmonary fibrosis.
- **Bronchocentric granulomatosis:**
  - ○ Clinical presentation includes cough, fever, chest pain, and hemoptysis.
  - ○ Two-thirds of patients do not have asthma.
  - ○ In nonasthmatic patients, there is an association with mycobacterial or fungal infections.

Gastrointestinal Disorders
- **Eosinophilic esophagitis (EE):**
  - ○ The presence of eosinophils in the esophagus is pathologic since normal esophagus should not contain eosinophils.[8]
  - ○ Gastroesophageal reflux (GERD) can also be associated with esophageal eosinophilia.
  - ○ EE is associated with both food and aero-allergens.[9]
  - ○ Eotaxin-3 is over-expressed in EE patients compared to the general population and may contribute to the pathogenesis of EE.[8]
  - ○ Patients present with vomiting, epigastric pain, dysphagia, and food impaction.
  - ○ It is more common in males.
  - ○ EE differs from GERD in the following ways: High prevalence of atopy, higher prevalence of food sensitization, commonly causes food impaction, normal pH in the esophagus, involvement of the proximal esophagus, higher level of eosinophils (>15/high-power field), and elevated eotaxin-3.[8]
- **Eosinophilic gastroenteritis:**
  - ○ Generally of idiopathic etiology, but like EE it is associated with food allergen sensitization.
  - ○ Increased peripheral blood IL-4 and IL-5.[10]
  - ○ It is associated with IgA deficiency.[8]
  - ○ Patients present with vomiting, abdominal pain, diarrhea, bloody stools, malabsorption, protein-losing enteropathy, and gastric outlet obstruction.
- **Eosinophilic colitis:**
  - ○ Generally not an IgE-mediated disease, possibly a T cell–driven process; offending protein triggers in the diet have been implicated in eosinophilic colitis of infants; pathogenesis is unclear.
  - ○ Bi modal age distribution with the first peak around 60 days of age and second peak around adolescence and early adulthood.[8]
  - ○ The presentation consists of diarrhea (may be bloody), weight loss, abdominal pain, and anorexia.
- **Other GI disorders** associated with varying degrees of tissue eosinophilia include Crohn's, disease, ulcerative colitis, GERD, and *Helicobacter pylori* infections.

Urinary Tract Disorders
- **Eosinophiluria** may be present in the following conditions:
  - ○ Drug-induced acute interstitial nephritis.
  - ○ Urinary tract infection, a common cause of eosinophiluria (minimal amount).
  - ○ Rapidly progressive and acute post-streptococcal glomerulonephritis.
  - ○ Eosinophilic prostatitis.
  - ○ Bladder cancer.
  - ○ Schistosomiasis with bladder involvement.

- **Eosinophilic cystitis:**
  - ○ Patients present with dysuria, hematuria, frequency, and suprapubic pain.
  - ○ It is more common in the pediatric population.
  - ○ Its etiology is unknown.
  - ○ Most patients have spontaneous resolution and an overall benign course, but the condition is associated with possibility of bladder carcinoma. Certain patients may develop renal failure and bladder destruction.[2]
- **Dialysis:**
  - ○ Patients on hemodialysis may develop mild eosinophilia.
  - ○ Patients on peritoneal dialysis may have episodic peritoneal eosinophilia and possibly peripheral blood eosinophilia that may be associated with infections.

Other
- **Hypoadrenalism:**
  - ○ Corticosteroids induce eosinophil apoptosis.
  - ○ Adrenal insufficiency in the form of Addison's disease, adrenal hemorrhage, hypopituitarism leads to decreased levels of endogenous corticosteroid production, thus, leading to peripheral blood eosinophilia.
- **Atheroembolic disease** may occur spontaneously or post-procedural.
- **Serosal irritation:**
  - ○ Dressler's syndrome (post-myocardial/post-pericardiotomy pericarditis).
  - ○ Eosinophilic pleural effusions.
  - ○ Eosinophilic ascites.
- **Primary immunodeficiency:** In patients with hyper-IgE syndrome, eosinophilia may be found in the peripheral blood, tissue, or sputum.
- **Transplant rejection:**
  - ○ Tissue infiltration of eosinophils is associated with acute allograft rejection for lung, kidney, and liver transplants.
  - ○ Eosinophilia of the blood and urine can be associated with both acute and chronic rejection of kidney allograft.
  - ○ With liver allograft rejection, peripheral and tissue eosinophilia may have diagnostic and prognostic utility as well as monitoring of the efficacy of rejection therapy.[2]
  - ○ Tissue eosinophilia may be present in cutaneous graft-versus-host disease.

Diagnostic Testing

- **General laboratory and diagnostic testing:**
  - ○ Comprehensive metabolic panel, absolute eosinophil count, and a chest radiograph.
  - ○ If a vasculitic syndrome is suspected, then antineutrophil cytoplasmic antibody (ANCA) and erythrocyte sedimentation rate (ESR) should be obtained.
  - ○ If parasitic infection is a possibility, then stool ova and parasite evaluation as well as parasitic antigens and serologic testing should be obtained.
- **Allergic disease:** If there are symptoms of allergic rhinitis or asthma, skin testing, and/or radioallergosorbent testing (RAST) for common aero-allergens can be performed.
- **Medication induced:** Careful medication history and documentation of time course of drug use and initiation is necessary for evaluation, especially any new drugs.
- **Infectious:**
  - ○ Stool studies are useful for enteric helminthes, but serologic testing is more sensitive and necessary for most infections.

- ○ Serologic testing and/or lung biopsy are indicated for coccidioidomycosis; skin biopsy may be helpful in disseminated infection.
- ○ Serum total IgE level, Aspergillus-specific IgE level, and skin testing for Aspergillus are used in ABPA.
- ○ HIV and HTLV-1 serologies.
- **Hypereosinophilic syndrome (HES):**
  - ○ **Myeloproliferative variant HES:**
    - Elevated vitamin B12 level, splenomegaly, cytogenetic abnormalities, and anemia may all be found.
    - Bone marrow biopsy may demonstrate extensive eosinophilic involvement or myelofibrosis.
    - May possess a fusion gene encoding FIP1L1/PDGFRA (platelet-derived growth factor alpha-receptor) protein expressing receptor kinase activity.
    - **FIP1L1/PDGFRA** may be detected by reverse transcription polymerase chain reaction (RT-PCR) or by fluorescence *in situ* hybridization (FISH) for the **CHIC-2 deletion.**
  - ○ **Lymphoproliferative variant HES:**
    - There may be clonal expansion of CD3-/CD4+ Th2-like lymphocytes producing IL-5.[2,11]
    - Detection is by flow cytometry as well as T-cell clonality analyses.
    - IgE level may be elevated.
  - ○ **Cardiac involvement testing:**
    - Troponin elevations may occur during in the acute setting.
    - Echocardiography may be useful in the later stages of disease.
    - Contrast-enhanced cardiac MRI has been shown to be sensitive in detection of cardiac involvement at all stages of disease.
- **Pulmonary:**
  - ○ The radiographic findings of pulmonary disorders associated with eosinophilia are presented in Table 18-2.
  - ○ **Chronic eosinophilic pneumonia:**
    - Peripheral blood eosinophilia in 90% of patients.[12]
    - IgE and ESR elevated in most patients.
    - Eosinophils and lymphocytes are found in bronchoalveolar lavage (BAL) fluid.
    - Pulmonary function tests (PFTs) may show diminished lung volumes, expiratory flow rates, and diffusing capacity.
  - ○ **Acute Eosinophilic pneumonia (AEP):**
    - Diffuse alveolar or alveolar–interstitial infiltrates are seen on chest radiographs.
    - Peripheral blood eosinophilia generally peaks around 7–9 days after presentation.
    - BAL eosinophils >25% or tissue eosinophilia seen on lung biopsy.
    - PFTs show decreased total lung capacity, decreased diffusing capacity, and small airway dysfunction, but generally normal forced expiratory volume at 1 second to forced vital capacity (FEV_1/FVC) ratio.
  - ○ **Churg–Strauss syndrome:**
    - Peripheral blood eosinophilia, increased ESR, and elevated serum IgE are usually seen.
    - A positive serum ANCA is seen in 40–60% of patients, usually perinuclear-ANCA.
  - ○ **Löffler's syndrome:**
    - Radiographs show unilateral or bilateral nonsegmental densities with indefinite borders; infiltrates are migratory and generally resolve over a few weeks.[2]

| TABLE 18-2 | RADIOGRAPHIC FEATURES OF PULMONARY DISORDERS WITH EOSINOPHILIA |

Syndrome	Radiographic features
Acute eosinophilic pneumonia	Diffuse bilateral alveolar or alveolar–interstitial infiltrates
ABPA	Pulmonary infiltrates with central bronchiectasis, "finger-in-glove" sign (medium size bronchi with mucus)
Bronchocentric granulomatosis	Focal mass or lobar consolidation with atelectasis
Chronic eosinophilic pneumonia	Described as a "photographic negative" of the appearance of pulmonary edema; peripheral infiltrates with no segmental or lobar restrictions in the outer lung zone with central sparing; nodular infiltration, bilateral consolidation, atelectasis, cavitation and pleural effusion; CT is more sensitive than plain chest radiography in detecting peripheral infiltrates; mediastinal lymphadenopathy may be present
Churg–Strauss syndrome	Patchy non-segmental consolidation on plain chest radiography; CT with airspace consolidation, bronchial wall thickening, ground-glass opacities, septal lines
Drug reaction	Consolidations with hilar adenopathy, pleural effusion, or reticulonodular densities
Hypereosinophilic syndrome	Patchy reticular densities, poorly defined nodules, and consolidation; cardiomegaly, pleural effusion
Löffler's syndrome	Unilateral/bilateral nonsegmental densities with ill-defined borders; migrating, transient infiltrates
Parasitic infection	Fine diffuse reticulonodular lesions often involving the lower lung zones
Pulmonary eosinophilic granuloma	Plain chest radiography shows reticulonodular infiltrates, cystic changes, honeycombing; CT shows cysts and nodules

ABPA, allergic bronchopulmonary aspergillosis.

- Peripheral blood eosinophilia may not be detectable in the early stage of pulmonary involvement but rises after several days of symptoms and returns to baseline after several weeks.
- Since it generally takes around 40 days for larva to mature into egg-producing adults, stool studies for helminthic ova are generally not diagnostic.
- Diagnosis is difficult to establish and requires finding larva in respiratory or gastric secretions.

- ○ **Tropical pulmonary eosinophilia:**
  - Peripheral blood eosinophilia, elevated IgG and IgE, and antifilarial antibodies are usually seen.
  - Eosinophilia is seen in BAL fluid.
  - Chest radiographs may show diffuse miliary lesions, consolidations, cavitations, and reticulonodular infiltrates.[2]
  - Lung biopsy reveals eosinophilic infiltration in the early stages and fibrosis in the later stages; microfilaria may be present.
- **Gastrointestinal:**
  - ○ **Eosinophilic esophagitis (EE):** Esophageal mucosal biopsy (via endoscopy), skin-prick testing for food and aero-allergens sensitization, and delayed skin patch testing are all potentially useful.
  - ○ **Eosinophilic gastroenteritis:** Endoscopy with biopsy and skin prick test to detect possible food allergies is necessary. Peripheral eosinophilia may be absent in one-quarter of patients.[8]
  - ○ **Eosinophilic colitis:** Colonoscopic biopsy, peripheral blood, and stool may all show eosinophilia.
- **Eosinophilic cystitis:**
  - ○ Cystoscopy reveals hyperemic mucosa with nodular or elevated regions.
  - ○ Biopsy demonstrates eosinophilic infiltrates, IgA and IgE plasma cells, and muscle necrosis. In more advanced disease fibrosis may be seen.
  - ○ Pelvic CT may be necessary to rule out other conditions.

TREATMENT

Allergic Diseases

Detailed discussions of the treatment of allergic rhinitis are found in Chapter 3 and for asthma in Chapter 4.

Medication Induced

- Drug therapy suspected of causing eosinophilia does not need to be stopped unless there is evidence of organ involvement.[13]
- Treatment then requires discontinuation of the offending medication.
- Time to resolution of eosinophilia after cessation of the drug is variable.

Infectious

Treatments for helminthic infections are beyond the scope of this chapter but include mebendazole, albendazole, ivermectin, pyrantel pamoate, and nitazoxanide.

Hypereosinophilic Syndrome

- Therapy for HES is not necessary without organ involvement.
- Initial treatment for patients without FIP1L1/PDGFRA mutation:
  - ○ Trial of 60 mg/day or 1 mg/kg/day of prednisone to determine if blood eosinophilia can be suppressed by steroids.
  - ○ Steroid dose can be tapered gradually for maintenance.[14]
  - ○ Prednisone-sensitive patients have a better prognosis.
- Imatinib should be used for the myeloproliferative variant, especially those with the FIP1L1/PDGFRA mutation.
  - ○ The dosage generally ranges from 100–400 mg/day.[2,15]
  - ○ Prospective studies show significant improvement in clinical and hematologic markers after therapy.[16,17]

- Second-line agents or steroid-sparing agents:
  - Hydroxyurea is the most frequently used second-line agent.[14]
    - Initial dose of 500–1,000 mg/day which can be increased to 2,000 mg/day.
    - Female patients need to be on contraception due to its teratogenic effects.
  - Interferon (IFN)-α:
    - INF-α is postulated to inhibit eosinophil proliferation as well as the inhibition of overall Th2 differentiation.[18]
    - Adverse effects include flu-like symptoms, depression, neuropathy, thyroid dysfunction, and elevated liver enzymes.
  - Anti-IL-5 monoclonal antibodies:
    - Preliminary results have shown some effectiveness in FIP1L1/PDGFRA-negative HES patients.[19,20]
    - Mepolizumab is currently only approved for case-by-case compassionate use.
    - Reslizumab is not yet approved for use.
  - Anti-CD52 monoclonal antibodies:
    - Target the surface protein CD52 that is expressed on eosinophils.
    - In one trial, 10 of 11 patients that were refractory to all other therapies treated with alemtuzumab achieved normalization of eosinophil counts in 2 weeks but most relapsed after 3 months.[21]
- Bone marrow transplantation has been done for HES but experience and evidence are fairly limited.

Pulmonary Disorders

- **Chronic eosinophilic pneumonia:**
  - Early treatment with corticosteroids is generally effective but disease can be recurrent and may become refractory to corticosteroids.
  - Peripheral eosinophilia decreases between 12–24 hours post initial therapy.[12]
  - Many patients achieve radiographic improvement in 60–72 hours after therapy initiation.
  - Most patients require more than 6 months of therapy.
  - Recurrences were seen in 58% of patients after cessation of steroids, so many patients might need long-term low-dose steroids.[12]
- **Acute eosinophilic pneumonia (AEP):**
  - Corticosteroids are very effective. Patients generally respond within 24–48 hours of high-dose therapy—tapering can be achieved over several weeks.
  - Prognosis is generally good with prompt treatment; disease is generally not recurrent.[2]
- **Churg–Strauss syndrome:**
  - Treatment generally consists of high-dose corticosteroids.
  - Cyclophosphamide for slow responders or patients who relapse during steroid taper.
- **Löffler's syndrome:** Acute symptoms generally resolve after 5–10 days after starting antihelminthic therapy.
- **Tropical pulmonary eosinophilia:** Diethylcarbamazine citrate is the appropriate antifilarial therapy.
- The treatment of **ABPA** is discussed in Chapter 4.
- **Drug- and toxin-induced eosinophilic lung disease** is treated with cessation of the drug or avoidance of the exposure. Corticosteroids can be used in more severe cases.

Gastrointestinal Disorders

- **Eosinophilic esophagitis** (EE):
  - The primary treatment is avoidance of specific food and aero-allergens. Elemental formulas (amino-acid based) diets have been shown to improve symptoms and reduce eosinophils.
  - Topical glucocorticoids must be swallowed to allow for deposition on the esophageal mucosa.[22]
  - Anti-IL-5 monoclonal antibodies (mepolizumab) is currently being studied for therapy in EE.
- **Eosinophilic gastroenteritis:**
  - Avoidance of food allergens is indicated and possibly the use of elemental formula diets.
  - Systemic and ingested topical corticosteroids (budesonide tablets designed to deliver medication to the ileum) may be helpful.
  - Anti-IL-5 and anti-IgE monoclonal antibodies are being studied.
- **Eosinophilic colitis:**
  - Treatment includes aminosalicylates and systemic and/or ingested topical corticosteroids.
  - Antimetabolite therapies such as azathioprine or 6-mercaptopurine can be used in steroid-refractory cases.
  - Surveillance with routine upper and lower endoscopies is recommended.
  - Prognosis of the adult onset disease is worse than the infantile type.[8]

Urinary Tract

- Corticosteroids may lead to improvement of eosinophilic cystitis.
- Acute interstitial nephritis is treated discontinuation of offending medication and steroids may be necessary in severe cases.

REFERENCES

1. Roufosse F, Weller PF. Practical approach to the patient with hypereosinophilia. *J Allergy Clin Immunol.* 2010;126:39–44.
2. Weller PF. Eosinophilia and eosinophil-related disorders. In: Adkinson NF Jr, Bochner BS, Busse WW, Holgate ST, Lemanske RF Jr, Simons FE, eds. *Middleton's Allergy Principles and Practice,* 7th ed. Philadelphia, PA: Mosby Elsevier, 2009:859–877.
3. Ruffing KA, Hoppes P, Blend D, et al. Eosinophils in urine revisited. *Clin Nephrol.* 1994; 41:163–166.
4. Wolf R, Matz H, Marcos B, et al. Drug rash with eosinophilia and systemic symptoms vs toxic epidermal necrolysis: the dilemma of classification. *Clin Dermatol.* 2005;23:311–334.
5. Junghans RP, Manning W, Safar M, et al. Biventricular cardiac thrombosis during interleukin-2 infusion. *N Engl J Med.* 2001;344:859–860.
6. Weller PF, Bubley GJ. The idiopathic hypereosinophilic syndrome. *Blood.* 1994;83:2759–2779.
7. Masi AT, Hunder GG, Lie JT, et al. The American College of Rheumatology 1990 criteria for the classification of Churg-Strauss syndrome (allergic granulomatosis and angiitis). *Arthritis Rheum.* 1990;33:1094–1100.
8. Rothenberg ME. Eosinophilic gastroenteropathies. In: Adkinson NF Jr, Bochner BS, Busse WW, Holgate ST, Lemanske RF Jr, Simons FE, eds. *Middleton's Allergy Principles and Practice,* 7th ed. Philadelphia, PA: Mosby Elsevier, 2009:879–891.
9. Onbasi K, Sin AZ, Doganavsargil B, et al. Eosinophil infiltration of the oesophageal mucosa in patients with pollen allergy during the season. *Clin Exp Allergy.* 2005;35:1423–1431.

10. Jaffe JS, James SP, Mullins GE, et al. Evidence for an abnormal profile of interleukin-4 (IL-4), IL-5, and gamma-interferon (gamma-IFN) in peripheral blood T cells from patients with allergic eosinophilic gastroenteritis. *J Clin Immunol.* 1994;14:299–309.
11. Roufosse F, Cogan E, Goldman M. Recent advances in pathogenesis and management of hypereosinophilic syndromes. *Allergy.* 2004;59:673–689.
12. Jederlinic PJ, Sicilian L, Gaensler EA. Chronic eosinophilic pneumonia. a report of 19 cases and a review of the literature. *Medicine.* 1988;67:154–162.
13. Olaison L, Belin L, Hogevik H, et al. Incidence of beta-lactam-induced delayed hypersensitivity and neutropenia during treatment of infective endocarditis. *Arch Intern Med.* 1999; 159:607–615.
14. Ogbogu PU, Bochner BS, Butterfield JH, et al. Hypereosinophilic syndrome: a multicenter, retrospective analysis of clinical characteristics and response to therapy. *J Allergy Clin Immunol.* 2009;124:1319–1325.
15. Baccarani M, Cilloni D, Rondoni M, et al. The efficacy of imatinib mesylate in patients with FIP1L1-PDGFRalpha-positive hypereosinophilic syndrome. Results of a multicenter prospective study. *Haematologica.* 2007;92:1173–1179.
16. Cools J, DeAngelo DJ, Gotlib J, et al. A tyrosine kinase created by fusion of the PDGFRA and FIP1L1 genes as therapeutic target of imatinib in idiopathic hypereosinophilic syndrome. *N Engl J Med.* 2003;348:1201–1214.
17. Jovanovic JV, Score J, Waghorn K, et al. Low-dose imatinib mesylate leads to rapid induction of major molecular responses and achievement of complete molecular remission in FIP1L1-PDGFRA-positive chronic eosinophilic leukemia. *Blood.* 2007;109:4635–4640.
18. Parronchi P, Mohapatra S, Sampognaro S, et al. Effects of interferon-alpha on cytokine profile, T cell receptor repertoire and peptide reactivity of human allergen-specific T cells. *Eur J Immunol.* 1996;26:697–703.
19. Rothenberg ME, Klion AD, Roufosse FE, et al. Treatment of patients with the hypereosinophilic syndrome with mepolizumab. *N Engl J Med.* 2008;358:1215–1228.
20. Garrett JK, Jameson SC, Thomson B, et al. Anti-interleukin-5 (mepolizumab) therapy for hypereosinophilic syndromes. *J Allergy Clin Immunol.* 2004;113:115–119.
21. Verstovsek S, Tefferi A, Kantarjian H, et al. Alemtuzumab therapy for hypereosinophilic syndrome and chronic eosinophilic leukemia. *Clin Cancer Res.* 2009;15:368–373.
22. Remedios M, Campbell C, Jones DM, et al. Eosinophilic esophagitis in adults: clinical, endoscopic, histologic findings, and response to treatment with fluticasone propionate. *Gastrointest Endosc.* 2006;63:3–12.

Mastocytosis

19

Bob Geng

GENERAL PRINCIPLES

- Mast cells play a central role in acquired immediate hypersensitivity reactions mediated through immunoglobulin E (IgE)-mediated release of histamine and other inflammatory mediators.
- Mastocytosis is the pathologic proliferation of mast cells resulting in uncontrolled release of inflammatory mediators causing both cutaneous and systemic clinical manifestations.[1]
- It is a rare disease that can occur at any age ranging from infancy to adulthood.

Classification

The classification of mastocytosis is presented in Table 19-1.[2]

Pathophysiology

- Mast cells are generally found in the gastrointestinal (GI) tract, respiratory tract, lymphoid tissues and skin. They are long-lived and do not generally circulate.
- Mature mast cells have cytoplasmic granules containing histamine and tryptase. Other components of granules include prostaglandin D2, leukotrienes C4, D4, E4, tumor necrosis factor (TNF)-α, platelet-activating factor (PAF), transforming growth factor (TGF)-β, endothelin, interleukin (IL)-3, IL-5, IL-6, and IL-16.[3,4]
- Symptoms associated with mastocytosis are **secondary to release of mast cell mediators** both within the tissues in which mast cells reside and distantly via circulation of those mediators.[1,3]
- Mast cells also display a vast array of antigens on their cell surface that serve as regulators of cell activation/recognition as well as receptors of various cytokines.
  - The proto-oncogene c-Kit encodes a transmembrane tyrosine kinase receptor for stem cell factor (SCF) that is significantly expressed in mast cells.
  - Point mutations of c-Kit such as D816V (most common), V560G, D816Y, D816F, D816H, E839K, F522C are associated with around 93% of all patients with systemic mastocytosis (SM).[3] The c-kit mutation is not detected in all mastocytosis.

DIAGNOSIS

Clinical Presentation

- **The vast majority (up to 90%) of adult and pediatric patients with mastocytosis have dermatologic involvement.** Affected areas usually include trunk and thighs sparing the face, palms, and soles.[1]
- **Cutaneous mastocytosis (CM)** can be classified by their characteristic presentation and appearance.

TABLE 19-1	CLASSIFICATION OF MASTOCYTOSIS

- Indolent mastocytosis
  - Cutaneous mastocytosis (CM) (infiltration of mast cells limited to the skin)
    - Urticaria pigmentosa (UP)
    - Diffuse cutaneous mastocytosis (DCM)
    - Mastocytoma of skin
  - Indolent systemic mastocytosis
- Systemic mastocytosis with associated clonal, hematologic nonmast cell lineage disease (SM-AHNMD)
- Aggressive systemic mastocytosis (ASM)
- Mast cell leukemia (MCL)

○ **Urticaria pigmentosa (UP):**
  - Small yellowish to reddish maculopapular lesions.
  - May present as nodules or plaques.
  - Spares the palms, soles, face, and scalp.
  - Rubbing can lead to urtication and erythema (Darier's sign).
  - Pruritus worsened by temperature change, local friction, hot beverages, spicy foods, and alcohol.
○ **Diffuse cutaneous mastocytosis (DCM):**
  - A rare condition.
  - No discrete lesions—diffuse infiltration of the dermis.
  - Erythroderma of all the skin.
  - Onset before 3 years old.
  - Skin is prematurely aged, thickened with a yellowish-brown color and peau d'orange texture.
○ Blisters can be associated with both UP and DCM in young children.
○ DCM can be associated with systemic disease and can lead to complications such as hypotension and GI bleeding.
○ In children, CM usually appears prior to the first year of life in around 80% of patients, but is usually not associated with systemic disease. Most will resolve spontaneously by puberty.[5]
○ **Solitary mastocytoma** (uncommon) presents as one reddish brown maculopapular lesion or nodule with a positive Darier's sign that often occurs during the first 3 months of life that usually resolves during childhood.[1]
○ **Telangiectasia macularis eruptive perstans (TMEP)** presents as telangiectatic macules that occur on tan-brown colored skin. Affects <1% of patients with mastocytosis. Usually only appears in adults, but there have been cases reported in the pediatric population.[1,3]
- **Systemic mastocytosis (SM)** clinical manifestations are the result of mast cell mediator release and mast cell infiltration into involved organs and tissues.
  ○ Owing to mast cell infiltration, organomegaly may be present (liver, spleen, and lymph nodes), and cytopenias can occur.
  ○ **Symptoms are nonspecific, but can include flushing, dyspepsia, diarrhea, recurrent syncope, recurrent anaphylaxis, bone pain, and fatigue.**
  ○ Patients with severe anaphylaxis to stings should be screened for mastocytosis
  ○ In aggressive forms of SM or in comorbid nonmast cell hematologic malignancies, symptoms of weight loss and fever may be present.

○ Mastocytosis needs to be considered in the evaluation of flushing syndromes especially with associated hypotension.

○ Systemic symptoms can occur in the absence of cutaneous symptoms.

○ SM is more common in adults than in children.

○ GI symptoms can be triggered or worsened by spicy foods, alcohol or stress, and is second most common compared to cutaneous symptoms.[3]

■ Abdominal pain, diarrhea, nausea, and vomiting occur.

■ One-third of SM patients experience malabsorption.

■ Caused by urticarial lesions in the GI tract, hypermotility, altered intestinal secretion, or peptic ulcer disease.

■ Hepatic involvement may result in elevated alkaline phosphatase and gamma-glutamyl transferase but rarely leads to serious disease.[3]

○ Splenic involvement usually results in trabecular, fibrotic thickening.

○ Musculoskeletal manifestations include osteoporosis, pathologic fractures, and nonspecific pains of unclear etiology. Bone discomfort usually involves the long bones and can be associated with pathologic fractures.

• **SM with associated clonal, hematologic nonmast cell lineage disease** (SM-AHNMD) can be seen in association with hypereosinophilic syndromes as well as other hematologic disorders.

• **Aggressive systemic mastocytosis** (ASM) and **mast cell leukemia** (MCL) are very rare and carry a poor prognosis.

Diagnostic Criteria

The World Health Organization diagnostic criteria for mastocytosis are presented in Table 19-2.[2]

Diagnostic Testing

Laboratories

• **Persistently elevated total serum tryptase level** (>20 ng/mL) is the most commonly used marker of SM.

• Elevated plasma/urine histamine or histamine metabolites (*N*-methylhistamine, methylimidazole acetic acid), urine prostaglandin D2 metabolites, plasma thromboxane B2, Il-6.

TABLE 19-2	WORLD HEALTH ORGANIZATION DIAGNOSTIC CRITERIA FOR MASTOCYTOSIS

• **Cutaneous mastocytosis:** Typical skin lesions and one of the following on skin biopsy
  • Focal dense (>15 mast cell per cluster) or diffuse mast cell infiltrates
  • c-Kit D816V mutation
• **Systemic mastocytosis:** One major and one minor or three minor criteria in bone marrow or organ biopsy
  • Major: Multifocal dense infiltrates of mast cell (>15 mast cells in aggregates)
  • Minor:
    • Mast cell infiltrates with greater than 25% spindle shaped, immature, or atypical morphology
    • Mutation in c-Kit D816V
    • CD2 and/or CD25 expression on CD117+ (encoded by c-kit) cells
    • Tryptase level in serum >20 ng/mL

- **Histamine level can be highly variable** between different individuals.
- Alkaline phosphatase and serum aminotransaminases can be elevated when there is hepatic involvement.
- Genetic testing for c-Kit mutation may be done.
- Urine level of 5-hydroxyindoleacetic acid and urine metanephrines to rule out carcinoid and pheochromocytomas as other possible causes of flushing and vascular instability.

Imaging
- Dual energy x-ray absorptiometry (DEXA), skeletal survey, and bone scans are often done for the evaluation of bone involvement. Osteoporosis is a common sequela of indolent systemic mastocytosis (ISM).
- When there is concern of liver or splenic involvement, abdominal ultrasound and/or CT may be done.

Diagnostic Procedures
- Suspected mastocytosis should be confirmed by tissue biopsy.
- **Skin biopsy** is usually preferred if the patient has cutaneous symptoms.
  - Histologically, mastocytosis characterized by **diffuse infiltration of mast cells in the dermis.**
  - Mast cells stain positive with toluidine blue or Wright–Giemsa as well as tryptase immunohistochemical analysis.
- **Bone marrow biopsy** can be helpful if the patient does not have cutaneous symptoms.
- A negative biopsy finding does not rule out disease since mast cells target organ effects could be secondary to mediator release rather than direct tissue infiltration.[1]

TREATMENT

Medications
- The mainstay of therapy is directed at control of symptoms from mediator release.
- **Antihistamines:**
  - H1 antagonists: Hydroxyzine, diphenhydramine, loratadine, fexofenadine, and cetirizine.
  - H2 antagonists: Ranitidine, cimetidine, and famotidine.
  - Can give one nonsedating antihistamine during the day and a more potent antihistamine at night.
- **Mast cell stabilizers:**
  - Gastric cromolyn formulations inhibit mast cell degranulation and are effective in reducing GI symptoms.[6]
  - Ketotifen is an antihistamine and a mast cell stabilizer that can be used but antihistamine properties are not more efficacious than hydroxyzine.[7]
- **Leukotriene modifying agents** may have some benefit.
- **Aspirin** can improve symptoms through blockade of prostaglandin synthesis but should be used with caution given the risk of triggering anaphylaxis.
- Patients with anaphylactoid reactions must be taught how to use self-administered intramuscular epinephrine injections (0.3 mg, 1:1,000) and must carry it with them at all times.
- **Oral glucocorticoids** can be most effective in treating malabsorption, ascites, hepatic fibrosis, and other GI symptoms but should be reserved for refractory disease or acute episodes.[8]

- Topical steroids may be used for cutaneous symptoms.
- **8-Methoxypsoralen with ultraviolet A phototherapy** (PUVA) can be used for cutaneous disease.[9]
- Surgical excision of a solitary lesion may also be an option.
- **Cytoreductive therapy** is only indicated for patients who present with target organ damage from aggressive systemic disease.
  - ○ **Interferon-α2b** is the first line agent.[3,10]
  - ○ **Cladribine** is a nucleoside analog that decreases mast cell burden.[11]
  - ○ **Tyrosine kinase inhibitors:**
    - Imatinib mesylate is approved by the FDA for ASM without D816V c-KIT mutation (only <10% of all cases). *In vitro* studies demonstrate that D816V c-KIT mutations confer resistance to imatinib.[1,3]
    - Imatinib should also be used for patients who have concomitant eosinophilia with the FIP1L1-PDGFRA fusion oncogene.[8,12]

Other Nonpharmacologic Therapies

- The first step in the therapeutic management of mastocytosis consists of patient counseling and education regarding the disease and **avoidance of triggers that may lead to MC degranulation.**
- Physical stimuli include intense exercise, excessive sunlight, friction, extreme temperatures, excessive pressure, and friction.[8]
- Emotional distress can trigger degranulation.[1,8]
- Multiple anesthetic agents have been implicated including lidocaine, succinylcholine, D-tubocurarine, metocurine, doxacurium, atracurium, mivacurium, rocuronium, thiopental, etomidate, enflurane, and isoflurane.[1]
- Other medications to consider include nonsteroidal anti-inflammatory drugs (NSAIDs), opiates, alcohol, vancomycin, α-blockers, thiamine, aspirin, amphotericin B, quinine, and polymyxin-B.[1,8]
- **Contrast agents** can provoke anaphylactoid reactions so all mastocytosis patients should be pre-medicated with steroids and antihistamines before receiving contrast. Gadolinium is not associated with MC degranulation.

OUTCOME/PROGNOSIS

- **CM has the best prognosis;** most children with isolated UP will have resolution by adulthood.[3,5]
- The prognosis of ISM is generally good and patients can have normal life expectancy. The probability of leukemic transformation is very low.[1,13]
- **The prognosis for ASM is generally poor** with median survival of 41 months.[1,13]
- For SM-AHNMD the prognosis is poor—median survival of 24 months, but this depends on the associated hematologic disorder.[1,13]
- MCL has a very poor prognosis, mean survival ranging from only 2–12 months.[3,13,14]

REFERENCES

1. Bains SN, Hsieh FH. Current approaches to the diagnosis and treatment of systemic mastocytosis. *Ann Allergy Asthma Immunol.* 2010;104:1–10.
2. Valent P, Akin C, Escribano L, et al. Standards and standardization in mastocytosis: consensus statements on diagnostics, treatment recommendations and response criteria. *Eur J Clin Invest.* 2007;37:435–453.

3. Metcalfe DD. Mastocytosis. In: Adkinson NF, Bochner BS, Busse WW, Holgate ST, Lemanske RF Jr, Simons FE, eds. *Middleton's Allergy Principles & Practice,* 7th ed. Philadelphia, PA: Mosby-Elsevier, 2009.

4. D'Ambrosio D, Akin C, Wu Y, et al. Gene expression analysis in mastocytosis reveals a highly consistent profile with candidate molecular markers. *J Allergy Clin Immunol.* 2003;112:1162–1170.

5. Kettelhut BV, Metcalfe DD. Pediatric mastocytosis. *J Invest Dermatol.* 1991;96:15S–18S.

6. Horan RF, Sheffer AL, Austen KF. Cormolyn sodium in the management of systemic mastocytosis. *J Allergy Clin Immunol.* 1990;85:852–855.

7. Kettelhut BV, Berkebile C, Bradley D, et al. A double-blind, placebo-controlled, crossover trial of ketotifen versus hydroxyzine in the treatment of pediatric mastocytosis. *J Allergy Clin Immunol.* 1989;83:866–870.

8. Wilson TM, Metcalfe DD, Robyn J. Treatment of systemic mastocytosis. *Immunol Allergy Clin North Am.* 2006;26:549–573.

9. Godt O, Proksch E, Streit V, et al. Short- and long-term effectiveness of oral and bath PUVA therapy in urticaria pigmentosa and systemic mastocytosis. *Dermatology.* 1997; 195:35–39.

10. Lim KH, Pardanani A, Butterfield JH, et al. Cytoreductive therapy in 108 adults with systemic mastocytosis: outcome analysis and response prediction during treatment with interferon-alpha, hydroxyurea, imatinib mesylate or 2-chlorodeoxyadenosine. *Am J Hematol.* 2009;84:790–794.

11. Kluin-Nelemans HC, Oldhoff JM, Van Doornaal JJ, et al. Cladribine therapy for systemic mastocytosis. *Blood.* 2003;102:4270–4276.

12. Ustun C, DeRemer DL, Atkin C. Thyrosine kinase inhibitors in the treatment of systemic mastocytosis. *Leuk Res.* 2011;35:1143–1152.

13. Pardanani A, Tefferi A. Systemic mastocytosis in adults: a review on prognosis and treatment based on 342 Mayo Clinic patients and current literature. *Curr Opin Hematol.* 2010;17:125–132.

14. Lim KH, Tefferi A, Lasho TL, et al. Systemic mastocytosis in 342 consecutive adults: survival studies and prognostic factors. *Blood.* 2009;113:5727–5736.

Primary Immunodeficiency Diseases

20

Sydney Leibel

GENERAL PRINCIPLES

- Primary immunodeficiencies (PIDs) are inherited disorders of immune system function that predispose affected individuals to **increased rate and severity of infection**, immune dysregulation with **autoimmune disease,** and **malignancy.**
- Most cases of PID are diagnosed during infancy and childhood, thus falling within the realm of pediatrics. However, a working knowledge of the classification and manifestations of PID and familiarity with the basic diagnostic and management strategies is beneficial for practitioners with patients of all ages.
- PIDs comprise more than 200 different disorders that affect the development, function, or both of the immune system.[1]

Classification

- PIDs are classified according to the component of the immune system that is primarily involved as adopted by the World Health Organization Scientific Group on PID.[2]
  - **Humoral** quantitative or qualitative defects in antibody production (50–60% of all PIDs).
  - Cell-mediated **T-cell deficiencies** (5–10% of all PIDs).
  - **Combined B- and T-cell deficiencies** (20–25% of all PIDs).
  - **Phagocytic cell or granulocyte disorders** are defects in migration or direct killing (10–15% of all PIDs).
  - **Complement deficiencies, defects in the innate immune system, and autoinflammatory syndromes** (<4% of all PIDs).
- Defects in adaptive immune responses include antibody deficiency syndromes and combined immunodeficiencies (CIDs).
- Defects of innate immunity comprise disorders of phagocytes, Toll-like receptor (TLR)-mediated signaling, and complement.
- A newly classified group of rare autoinflammatory conditions with associated immunodeficiency.
- **A genetic defect has been identified for many PIDs.** The majority are X-linked or autosomal recessive.

Epidemiology

- **The most common PID is immunoglobulin A (IgA) deficiency.** It has a reported frequency of 1 in 333 among some blood donors.[3]
- All other forms of PID are rare and have an overall prevalence of approximately 1:10,000 live births.
- A much higher rate is observed among populations with high consanguinity rates or among genetically isolated populations.

DIAGNOSIS

Clinical Presentation

History

- **A history of recurrent, chronic, prolonged, complicated, severe, or opportunistic infections in a patient without known secondary immunodeficiency** (i.e., malignancy, HIV/AIDS, immunosuppressive therapy, malnutrition) should cause prompt consideration for PID.[4]
- Historical clues to the presence of PID are given in Table 20-1.
- Given the rarity of PID and the cost and potential morbidity associated with immunologic testing, a history compatible with PID is an absolute prerequisite for embarking on a laboratory workup to confirm a clinical diagnosis of PID.
- Clinical presentation and the etiologic agents involved are the best clues to the class of PIDs suspected (Table 20-2).
- Types and patterns of infection:
  - **Recurrent or chronic** infections: An often-cited guideline is **>6–8 upper respiratory tract infections (URIs) per year in the first decade of life or more than one episode of pneumonia per decade in adults.** It is important to note, however, that children exposed to frequent daycare and/or tobacco smoke may have up to 10 URIs per year. Also, any serious infection occurring twice in a child or once in an adult should raise suspicion of presence of PID.
  - **Prolonged duration** of infections.
  - **Severe or complicated infections:** For example, severe varicella complicated by pneumonia or hepatitis or bronchiectasis.
  - **Infection with an opportunistic** organism: For example, *Pneumocystis jirovecii* pneumonia, *Pseudomonas aeruginosa*, *Cryptococcus neoformans* (in the absence of HIV/AIDS).

TABLE 20-1	HISTORICAL CLUES TO PRESENCE OF PRIMARY IMMUNODEFICIENCY DISEASES

Recurrent, chronic, or severe sinopulmonary (including otic) infections
Complicated sinopulmonary/otic infections
Recurrent or severe infections with encapsulated bacteria (pneumonia, meningitis, sepsis)
Requirement of repeated courses of antibiotics
Opportunistic infections
Failure to thrive, wasting
Recurrent or chronic diarrhea, malabsorption
Adverse reaction to live-virus immunization
Adverse reaction to blood or plasma transfusions (graft-vs-host)
Recurrent infections of skin
Recurrent deep-seeded or organ abscesses
Recurrent periodontitis
Recurrent neisserial infections
Recurrent autoimmune phenomena
Delayed separation of umbilical cord

TABLE 20-2	COMMON PRESENTATIONS AND INFECTIOUS AGENTS CLASSIFIED BY PRIMARY IMMUNODEFICIENCY DISEASE SUBTYPE

Clinical presentation	Etiologic agent
Antibody deficiencies	
Sinusitis	*Streptococcus pneumoniae*
Pneumonia	*Haemophilus influenza*
Pharyngitis	*Moraxella catarrhalis*
Otitis	*Neisseria meningitides*
Meningitis	*Staphylococcus aureus*
Bacteremia	*Pseudomonas spp.*
Encephalitis (enteroviral)	Enterovirus (echovirus and poliovirus)
Colitis (giardiasis)	Rotavirus
	Giardia lamblia
	Cryptosporidium
	Mycoplasma (including *Ureaplasma urealyctium*)
Combined T- and B-cell deficiencies	
Opportunistic infections	*Mycobacterium tuberculosis*
Failure to thrive	*Mycobacterium avium intracellulare*
Diarrhea	*Listeria monocytogenes*
Dermatitis	*Pneumocystis jirovecii*
Sepsis	*Toxoplasma gondii*
	Candida albicans
	Nocardia asteroides
	Isospora belli
	Cryptosporidium hominis
	Cytomegalovirus
	Herpes simplex
	Herpes zoster
	Epstein–Barr virus
Phagocytic cell disorders	
Invasive skin infections/abscesses	*S. aureus*
Focal abscesses	*Pseudomonas cepacia*
Poor wound healing	*Salmonella typhimurium*
Lymphadenitis	*Serratia typhimurium*
Periodontitis	*Serratia marcescens*
	Klebsiella spp.
	Escherichia coli
	Mycobacterium fortuitum
	Aspergillus spp.
	C. albicans
	Actinomyces spp.
Complement deficiencies	
Pyogenic infections	*N. meningitides*
C5–C9 deficiencies	*Neisseria gonorrhea*
C3 Deficiencies	*S. pneumoniae*
Innate immune system	
Pyogenic infections	*S. pneumoniae*
Viral infections	*S. aureus*
	M. fortuitum
	Herpes simplex
	Human papilloma virus

- The presence of certain features or constellations of signs should prompt suspicion of PID, such as:
  - ○ Cardiac disease, micrognathia, and hypocalcemia (DiGeorge syndrome).
  - ○ Thrombocytopenia and eczema (Wiskott–Aldrich syndrome).
  - ○ Hypohidrosis, dental anomalies, alopecia (NEMO [nuclear factor-κ-B essential modulator] mutation, hypohidrotic ectodermal dysplasia with immunodeficiency).
  - ○ Ataxia plus oculocutaneous telangiectasias (ataxia-telangiectasia syndrome).
- Elements of the history that can help in the diagnosis are:
  - ○ Family member with documented PID or recurrent infections.
  - ○ Unexplained early infant deaths.
  - ○ Autoimmune disease.
  - ○ Consanguinity.

Physical Examination

The physical examination findings of PIDs are presented in Table 20-3.

TABLE 20-3	PHYSICAL EXAMINATION FINDINGS IN PRIMARY IMMUNODEFICIENCY DISEASE
Finding	**Association**
Failure to thrive	T-cell deficiencies
Atypical facies	DiGeorge syndrome, hyper-IgE syndrome
Mucocutaneous candidiasis	Combined T- and B-cell deficiencies; Wiskott–Aldrich syndrome
Cutaneous ulcers	Severe T-cell deficiencies; hyper-IgM syndrome
Cutaneous abscesses	Phagocyte deficiencies; hyper-IgE syndrome
Atopic dermatitis	Wiskott–Aldrich syndrome; hyper-IgE syndrome; hypogammaglobulinemia
Telangiectasias (eye involvement)	Ataxia-telangiectasia syndrome
Albinism (oculocutaneous)	Chediak–Higashi syndrome
Clubbing	Various
Recurrent otitis media, sinusitis	Various
Periodontitis	Phagocyte deficiencies
Small or absent tonsilar, adenoidal, peripheral lymph nodes	T-cell and B-cell deficiencies
Lymphadenopathy, splenomegaly, and hepatomegaly	Omenn syndrome; hyper-IgM syndrome, CVID, ALPS
Arthritis, autoimmunity (lupus)	Antibody deficiencies, complement deficiencies
Delayed umbilical cord detachment	Leukocyte adhesion defects
Recurrent fever, urticaria, inflammatory conditions (uveitis, myositis, serositis)	Autoinflammatory syndromes

IgM, immunoglobulin M; CVID, common variable immune deficiency; ALPS, autoimmune lymphoproliferative syndrome.

Diagnostic Testing

Laboratories

- A **complete blood count (CBC) with differential** should be ordered in all cases of suspected immunodeficiency.
  - A CBC may indicate lymphopenia; however, a normal WBC does not exclude lymphopenia. This value consists of both lymphocytes and granulocytes, which is why a differential is required.
  - Total lymphocyte count should be >1,200 cells/μL in adults, >3,000 cells/μL in infants.
  - Because T cells make up approximately 75% of the total lymphocyte count, lymphopenia typically implies a decreased number of T cells.
  - Alternatively, **leukocytosis** may be present, which is a sign of leukocyte adhesion defects.
  - **Eosinophilia** (>1.5 × 10^9/L) is present in hyper-IgE syndrome.
  - **Thrombocytopenia** (<70,000/μL) with **small platelets** is seen in Wiskott–Aldrich syndrome.
- **Rule our cystic fibrosis and immotile cilia syndrome.**
  - Cystic fibrosis presents with recurrent episodes of bronchitis, sinusitis, and pneumonia and is associated with malnutrition, failure to thrive, and steatorrhea.
  - If features of the disease are present, a **sweat chloride** screening test should be performed.
    - >60 mEq/L is abnormal in children; >80 mEq/L in adults.
    - Sensitivity of this test is 80–85%.
  - If the clinical suspicion is high, but the sweat test is negative or equivocal, genetic testing for **cystic fibrosis transmembrane regulator** (CFTR) gene mutations should be performed.
  - Immotile cilia syndrome is characterized as an autosomal recessive condition with recurrent upper and lower respiratory infections and bronchiectasis.
- Consider **HIV infection** in those with risk factors.
  - HIV antibodies are usually sufficient; however, in those with decreased or absent immunoglobulin response obtaining and HIV viral load is recommend.
- **Quantitative immunoglobulins** (IgG, IgA, IgM, IgE) should be interpreted according to age-related standards (see Appendix B, Table B-3). Hypogammaglobulinemia is defined by immunoglobulin levels two standard deviations below the mean for age.
- **Saline isohemagglutinins** (anti-A, anti-B) are used to assess IgM function.
  - Isohemagglutinins are normally lacking in persons with blood type AB.
  - Unreliable in infants <6 months of age or in individuals who have received intravenous or subcutaneous γ globulin within 30 days.
- **Antibody response to immunization** is a functional test for the immune system. Pre- and post-immunization antibody titers should be measured 3–4 weeks apart.
  - **Pneumococcal polysaccharide vaccination** (e.g., Pneumovax 23) is more useful for impaired antibody production than protein-conjugated polysaccharide vaccines (e.g., Hib, tetanus, or Hib-diphtheria conjugates), though it is advised to measure responses to both polysaccharide and protein-conjugated vaccines (see Appendix B, Table B-5 for reference values).
  - Antibody responses to carbohydrate antigens are typically poor in children <2 years old.
  - Booster immunizations with repeat titers 3–4 weeks later may be required in children and in adults with long intervals since previous vaccination.

- **Delayed-type hypersensitivity (DTH)** skin tests are functional tests of cell-mediated immunity.
  - Only four antigens intended for assessing a person's ability to elicit a DTH response have been standardized for this use by the Mantoux procedure: **Tuberculin, coccidioidin, histoplasmin, and mumps.**
  - Only a very small proportion of the population will react to tuberculin.
  - Sensitivity to coccidioidin and histoplasmin is restricted to endemic regions.
  - In large trials conducted by the army medical centers, mumps, Candida, and tetanus toxoid produced the highest proportion of positive skin tests, although only mumps is standardized for anergy testing.
- **T- and B-lymphocyte subsets** (CD3, CD4, CD8, CD19, CD16, and CD56) and *in vitro* **responses to mitogens** should be measured by a laboratory that provides age-matched normal control values (see Appendix B, Table B-6).
- **Laboratory evaluation for specific immunodeficiencies:**
  - **Complement deficiency:** Total hemolytic complement (CH50) approaches zero in individuals with deficiency of any of the classic complement pathway components except C9. C3 and C4 can be used as a screening test.
  - **Phagocyte deficiency:** Flow cytometry assay using dihydrorhodamine (DHR) oxidation or the nitroblue tetrazolium test to demonstrate failure of the normal respiratory burst in chronic granulomatous disease.
  - **DiGeorge syndrome:** Fluorescent *in situ* hybridization (FISH) for the 22q11 mutation that 90% of affected patients have.
  - Hyper IgE syndrome: Signal transducer and activator of transcription 3 (**STAT3**) mutation is the most common mutation in the autosomal dominant form of the disease.

Selected Primary Immunodeficiency Diseases

It is beyond the scope of this book to provide an in-depth review of the clinical and laboratory features of PID. Table 20-4 summarizes the immunologic profile and genetic defects associated with PIDs.[1]

X-linked Severe Combined Immunodeficiency

- X-linked SCID is the most common form of severe combined immunodeficiency (50–60%).[5]
- Affected infants present within the first few months with frequent episodes of diarrhea, pneumonia, otitis media, cutaneous infections, and sepsis.
- The disease is characterized by **profound T- and B-cell lymphopenia.** There is an absence of T-cell proliferation, **serum immunoglobulins are low or absent,** and there is minimal antibody response to vaccination.
- Physical examination may reveal small or absent lymph nodes, tonsils, and adenoids. Growth may be normal at first but extreme wasting usually develops. An absent thymic shadow may be noticed on chest radiograph.
- X-linked SCID is a **pediatric medical emergency.** Treatment includes empiric antimicrobial coverage, intravenous immunoglobulin (IVIG), and stem cell transplant. Bone marrow or other stem cell reconstitution is a first-line, specific therapy for almost all forms of SCID. Patients who are well nourished, uninfected, and younger than 6 months prior to transplantation have the best outcomes.
- Without stem cell reconstitution, it is rare for a patient with SCID to survive.

TABLE 20-4 SUMMARY OF SELECTED IMMUNOLOGIC PROFILE AND GENETIC DEFECTS ASSOCIATED WITH PID

General category	Disorder	T-cell levels	B-cell levels	Ig levels	Defect
Combined T- and B-cell deficiencies	Gamma chain deficiency	Low	Normal to high	Low	Defect in gamma chain of receptors for IL-2, IL-4, IL-7, IL-9, IL-15
	Jak3 kinase deficiency	Low	Normal to high	Low	Jak3 intracellular signaling defect
	Adenosine deaminase deficiency	Progressive decrease	Progressive decrease	Low	Build-up of toxic purine pathway intermediated in lymphocytes
	Purine nucleoside phosphorylase deficiency	Progressive decrease	Normal	Normal or low	Build-up of toxic purine pathway intermediates in T lymphocytes
	MHC II deficiency	Low CD4	Normal	Normal or low	Mutations in transcription factors for MHC II gene expression
	Zap-70 kinase deficiency	Low CD8	Normal	Normal	Thymocyte intracellular kinase defect, blocked maturation of T cells
	Recombinase activating gene (RAG1, RAG2) deficiency	Low	Low	Low	T-cell and B-cell receptor rearrangement failure, blocked lymphocyte development
	Reticular dysgenesis	Low	Low	Low	Unknown bone marrow stem cell defect
	Omenn syndrome	Low	Low	Low	Missense mutation in RAG1 or RAG2 resulting in partial V-D-J recombination activity

	DiGeorge syndrome	Normal to low	Normal	Normal to low	Embryologic defect of thymic development; variably associated defects of heart, parathyroid, facial development
Antibody deficiencies	X-linked agammaglobulinemia	Normal	Very low (<2%) to absent	Low to absent	Defect of B-cell specific Bruton tyrosine kinase
	Autosomal recessive agammaglobulinemia	Normal	Very low to absent	Low to absent	Defects in components of B-cell receptor chain, chain, IgA, IgB, BLNK
	X-linked hyper-IgM syndrome	Normal	Normal	Normal to high IgM, low IgA and IgG	Defect in CD40 ligand causing failure of B-cell isotype switch
	IgA deficiency and IgG subclass deficiency	Normal	Normal	One or more immunoglobulin types low	Unknown defects in B-cell isotype expression, IgG subclass deficiencies associated with immunoglobulin heavy or light chain gene deletions
	Common variable immunodeficiency	Normal	Normal or low	Low (variable)	Unknown late-onset variable defects in B and T-cell function and regulation
	Transient hypo-gammaglobulinemia of infancy	Normal	Normal	Low IgG, low or normal IgA, normal IgM	Delayed onset of IgG synthesis; cause unknown
Other well-defined syndromes	Wiskott–Aldrich syndrome	Normal to low	Normal	Normal (some low IgM)	Defect in *WASP* gene involved in cytoskeleton, sparse small platelets, eczema

(continued)

TABLE 20-4 SUMMARY OF SELECTED IMMUNOLOGIC PROFILE AND GENETIC DEFECTS ASSOCIATED WITH PID (continued)

General category	Disorder	T-cell levels	B-cell levels	Ig levels	Defect
	Ataxia telangectasia	Normal	Normal	Low	DNA repair defect in *AATM* gene; *ataxia, progressive neurodegeneration; cancer;* radiation sensitivity
	Bloom syndrome	Normal	Normal	Selective IgM deficiency	DNA repair defect in *BLM* gene, progressive neurodegeneration, cancer, radiation sensitivity
	Hyper IgE syndrome	Normal	Normal	High IgE	*STAT3* mutation most common AD inheritance, susceptibility to cutaneous boils and lung abscesses
	X-linked lymphoproliferative syndrome	Normal	Normal	Progressive loss	Failure to resolve Epstein–Barr virus infections associated with lymphoproliferation and, ultimately, hypogammaglobulinemia
	Cartilage-hair hypoplasia	Low	Normal	Normal	Short-limbed dwarfism associated with cellular immunodeficiency
	APCED autoimmune polyendocrinopathy with candidiasis and ectodermal dystrophy	Normal	Normal	Normal	Defects in *AIRE*, encoding a transcription regulator needed to establish thymic self-tolerance. Autoimmunity and candidiasis.

	Lack of CD4 CD25 FOXP3 regulatory T cells	Normal	Elevated IgE, IgA	
IPEX immune dysregulation, polyendocrinopathy, enteropathy (X-linked)	Lack of CD4 CD25 FOXP3 regulatory T cells	Normal	Elevated IgE, IgA	Defect in *FOXP3*, encoding a T cell transcription factor. Autoimmunity and eczema.
Phagocyte disorders				
Chronic granulomatous disease	Normal	Normal	Normal	Impaired killing of organisms due to defects of neutrophil cytochrome oxidase system
Leukocyte adhesion deficiency	Normal	Normal	Normal	Defects of leukocyte surface proteins required for adhesion, migration, and phagocytosis (CD18-LAD type I)
Chediak–Higashi syndrome	Normal	Normal	Normal	Defect in *CHM* gene causing faulty lysosomal assembly, giant cytoplasmic granules, impaired neutrophil function

(continued)

TABLE 20-4 SUMMARY OF SELECTED IMMUNOLOGIC PROFILE AND GENETIC DEFECTS ASSOCIATED WITH PID (continued)

General category	Disorder	T-cell levels	B-cell levels	Ig levels	Defect
Complement disorder	Individual component deficiencies	Normal	Normal	Normal	C1, C2, C4, and C3 deficiencies associated with autoimmunity and pyogenic infections. C5–9 and properdin deficiencies associated with recurrent neisserial infections.
Defects in innate immunity	Anhidrotic ectodermal dysplasia with immunodeficiency	Normal	Normal	Normal-poor function	Mutations of NEMO (IKBKG), a modulator of NF-kB activation. Anhidrotic ectodermal dysplasia and specific antibody deficiency (poor polysaccharide response).
Autoinflammatory disorders	Periodic Mediterranean fever	Normal	Normal	Normal	Mutation of MEFV. Decreased pyrin production, recurrent fever, serositis and inflammation responsive to colchicines. Predisposes to vasculitis and inflammatory bowel disease

PID, primary immunodeficiency.

IgA Deficiency

- IgA deficiency is **the most common PID**, affecting 1:300–1:700 individuals.
- Diagnostic criteria for selective IgA deficiency include a **serum IgA level <10 mg/dL** (or below the level of detection) with normal levels of other immunoglobulin classes and normal cellular immunity. Vaccine responses are also usually normal.
- The disease is more prevalent among persons with recurrent infections, allergy, autoimmune disorders, and certain GI disorders like celiac disease.
- Clinical expression of IgA deficiency ranges from recurrent sinopulmonary or GI infections to no symptoms.
- IgA deficiency is difficult to diagnosis prior to the age of 2 given the natural course of IgA antibody production (see Table 20-4).[6]
- An estimated one-third of patients with IgA deficiency have **serum IgE antibodies to IgA** that can cause anaphylaxis during transfusion of blood products or IVIG.
- Treatment of IgA deficiency is supportive, with antimicrobial therapy as needed and treatment of autoimmune disorders. A small portion of IgA deficiency patients go on to develop CVID, thus serum immunoglobulins should be monitored over time.

Common Variable Immunodeficiency

- Common variable immunodeficiency is a **heterogeneous disorder characterized by recurrent bacterial infections, severe hypogammaglobulinemia, and diminished antibody responses.** It typically affects older children and adults and is classically diagnosed during the second and third decade of life.
- Clinical manifestations include recurrent **sinopulmonary infections, bronchiectasis, malabsorption, and diarrhea** (usually associated with *Giardia lamblia* infection). Some patients have respiratory tract colonization with *Mycoplasma* or *Ureaplasma* organisms.
- **Autoimmune disease** may also be present (e.g., pernicious anemia, hemolytic anemia, polyarticular arthritis, lupus-like syndromes).
- There is also an increased risk of **lymphoreticular malignancy.**[7]
- Physical examination may reveal diminished lymph nodes and tonsilar tissue, though there may be signs of lymphoid hypertrophy in the form of lymphadenopathy and/or splenomegaly.
- Serum IgG and IgA levels are usually low and most antibody responses are poor or absent. B-cell subpopulation is typically normal.
- Treatment is supportive, including IVIG.

TREATMENT

- Pathogen avoidance is crucially important.
- Early and judicious use of **empiric antibiotics** followed by culture-directed specific antibiotic treatment.
- Consider fungal, mycobacterial, viral, or protozoan pathogens early in management if infections is refractory to antibiotics.
- **IVIG** (or subcutaneous IG) is paramount in the management of PID due to antibody deficiency.
  - Mechanism of action. Commercially available preparations contain IgG antibodies (pooled from >3,000 donors) in concentrations sufficient to serve as replacement for IgG as well as trace amounts of IgA and IgM.
  - Recommended starting dosage is **400–500 mg/kg every month.**

○ Trough serum IgG level (target >500 mg/dL or higher if bronchiectasis present) measured 4 weeks after IVIG infusion are used to guide dosage and frequency.

○ The subcutaneous route can be used in stabilized patients for **weekly home use.**

○ Adverse effects include fever, nausea, vomiting, and back pain. Severe **anaphylactic reactions rarely occur** (possibly due to trace amounts of IgA in the IVIG).

○ Aseptic meningitis and hemolytic anemia are also rare complications. Treatment of aseptic meningitis treatment is supportive. Evidence in lacking to support use of high dose steroids.

- **Stem cell transplantation** has been used to correct the underlying immune defects in SCID, chronic granulomatous disease, hyper-IgM syndrome, and Wiskott–Aldrich syndrome.

- **Gene therapy and replacement enzyme therapy** have been utilized in SCID and may have further use in complement deficiency.

- Parents of a child with diagnosed immunodeficiency may desire evaluation to see if one or both parents carry the defect, in order to plan for future childbearing. In X-linked diseases this can be accomplished by x-chromosome inactivation analysis.

- **Blood products** may elicit life-threatening graft-vs-host disease in patients with cellular immunodeficiency and anaphylaxis in those with antibody deficiency.

- **Live virus vaccines** (e.g., measles/mumps/rubella, varicella, rotavirus) **should not be given** to patients with PID or their family members.

REFERENCES

1. Notarangelo LD. Primary immunodeficiencies. *J Allergy Clin Immunol.* 2010;125:S182–S194.
2. Rezaei N, Bonilla FA, Sullivan KE, et al. An introduction to primary immunodeficiency diseases. In: Rezaei N, Notarangelo LD, Aghamohammadi A, eds. *Primary Immunodeficiency Diseases: Definition, Diagnosis, and Management.* Berlin: Springer, 2008:1–29.
3. Clark JA, Callicoat PA, Brenner NA. Selective IgA deficiency in blood donors. *Am J Clin Pathol.* 1983;80:210–213.
4. Buckley RH. Primary immunodeficiency disease. In: Adkinson NF, Bochner BS, Busse WW, Holgate ST, Lemanske RF Jr, Simons FE, eds. *Middleton's Allergy Principles and Practice,* 7th ed. Philadelphia, PA: Elsevier Inc., 2009:1027–1049.
5. Buckley RH. Molecular defects in human severe combined immunodeficiency and approaches to immune reconstitution. *Annu Rev Immunol.* 2004;22:625–655.
6. Janeway CA, Murphy K, Travers T, et al. *Janeway Immunobiology Figure 12–10,* 7th ed. New York, NY: Garland Science, 2008.
7. Cunningham-Rundles C, Cooper DL, Duffy TP. Lymphomas of mucosal-associated lymphoid tissue in common variable immunodeficiency. *Am J Hematol.* 2002;69:171–178.

Allergen Immunotherapy

21

James A. Tarbox

GENERAL PRINCIPLES

- Allergen immunotherapy (IT) is used in allergic rhinitis, allergic asthma, stinging-insect hypersensitivity, and atopic dermatitis if associated with aeroallergen sensitivity.
- Standardized extracts should be used when available.
- **IT should only be performed by a specialist trained in allergy and immunology.**
- Treatment needs to be tailored for the individual, with appropriate concentrations of allergens for approximately 3–5 years duration.

Definition

IT is the administration of increasing doses of allergen extract to alleviate symptoms associated with the causative allergen.

Pathophysiology

- The mechanism of action of IT is complex and not yet well understood.
- One current theory is that introduction of the allergen results in immune modulation of the immune system that shifts the T-cell phenotype from a T_H2 toward a T_H1 predominance (Fig. 21-1).[1]
- T-regulatory cells producing interleukin (IL)-10 and transforming growth factor (TGF)-β are increased in successful IT.[2]
- Studies have shown that IT leads to:
  - Blunting of the usual seasonal rise in IgE antibodies over time.
  - Increase in serum IgA and IgG antibodies with change in subclasses (increased IgG1 and IgG4).
  - Down-regulation of the cellular and inflammatory mediators of allergic response.
  - Decrease in platelet-activating factor and histamine-releasing factor levels.
  - Down-regulation of the low-affinity IgE receptor (Fcε RII).
  - Decrease in mast cell and eosinophil numbers in secretions.
  - Up-regulation of the counter-regulatory cytokines expressed by T_H1 phenotype.

TREATMENT

Efficacy

- The clinical efficacy of IT in allergic rhinitis has been well documented, and IT has been shown to improve symptoms, reduce medications, and provide long-term benefits even after cessation of therapy.[3–5]

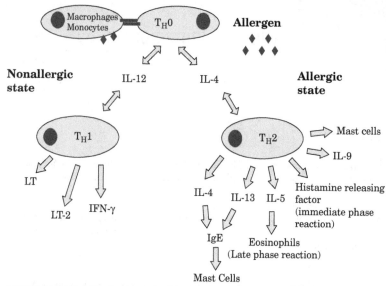

FIGURE 21-1 Simplified schematic diagram of the T$_H$1 and T$_H$2 paradigm in allergic diseases. The T$_H$2 profile is associated with the allergic state and humoral immune responses, whereas the T$_H$1 profile is associated with cellular responses and a down-regulation in allergic responses. Immunotherapy is thought to shift the T-cell phenotype from T$_H$2 toward T$_H$1. A representation of cytokines involved in this is shown. DC, dendritic cell; IL, interleukin; INF, interferon; T$_H$0,undifferentiated T-helper cell; TNF, tumor necrosis factor.

- Allergen-specific IT has the potential to alter the natural course of allergic disease.[6]
- IT improves asthma symptoms, decreases use of asthma medications, and reduces bronchial hyper-reactivity.[7]
- Long-term benefits of >12 years after discontinuation of therapy in patients with allergic rhinitis have been documented.[8,9]
- The quality of the extract used for successful IT is critical.[10] The World Health Organization (WHO) has endorsed the use of standardized extracts whenever available in IT.[11]
- Achieving optimal target doses of the causative allergen is also critical for IT to be successful.
- Table 21-1 provides recommended maintenance doses set forth by the Joint Task Force for allergen IT practice parameters.[12]

Indications

- IT is indicated for allergic rhinitis/conjunctivitis, allergic reactions to stinging insects, allergic asthma, and atopic dermatitis resulting from sensitivity to aeroallergens.
- It is **not indicated for food or drug allergy, urticaria, or angioedema.**[13]
- Criteria for initiating IT:

TABLE 21-1	ALLERGEN IMMUNOTHERAPY RECOMMENDED MAINTENANCE DOSES		
Allergen	Dose, standardized units	Dose, major allergen	Maintenance concentrate, wt/vol[a]
Dermatophagoides pteronyssinus	600 AU	7–12 µg, Der p1	NA
Dermatophagoides farinae	2,000 AU	10 µg, Der f1	NA
Cat	2,000–3,000 BAU	11–17 µg, Fel d1	NA
Grass (e.g., timothy)	4,000 BAU	7 µg, Phl p5	NA
Short ragweed (standardized)	NA	6–24 µg, Amb a1	1:100–1:30
Other pollen (nonstandardized)	NA	ND	1:100–1:30
Fungi/mold (nonstandardized)	NA	ND	1:100–1:50

AU, allergy unit; BAU, bioequivalent allergy unit; NA, not applicable; ND, not determined.
[a]Based on a maintenance injection of 0.5 mL.

Reprinted with permission from: Joint Task Force on Practice Parameters. Allergen immunotherapy: a practice parameter. American Academy of Allergy, Asthma and Immunology. American College of Allergy, Asthma and Immunology. *Ann Allergy Asthma Immunol.* 2003;90:1–40.

- ○ **Demonstration that the disease is IgE-mediated**—epicutaneous skin test is the preferred method.
- ○ **Pharmacotherapy** (e.g., antihistamines, decongestants, leukotriene modulators, topical corticosteroids) **and/or allergen avoidance have not successfully controlled symptoms.**
- Indications for IT (any one of the following):
  - ○ Insufficient symptom control with antihistamines, decongestants, topical corticosteroids, and/or leukotriene modulators.
  - ○ Undesirable side effects of pharmacotherapy.
  - ○ Desire to avoid or reduce long-term pharmacologic treatment.
  - ○ Patients with allergic asthma with mild-to-moderate disease (forced expiratory volume in 1 second [FEV_1] >70% of predicted) on adequate pharmacologic treatment.
  - ○ Hypersensitivity to *Hymenoptera* or fire ants and at risk for anaphylaxis.

Allergic Rhinitis
Commonly cited reasons for initiating IT in allergic rhinitis[11]:
- To prevent symptoms and improve quality of life.
- To reduce ongoing expenses for noncurative medication.
- To reduce side effects of antihistamines and decongestants.

- To reduce development/aggravation of allergic asthma.
- To reduce comorbidity due to recurrent sinusitis/otitis.
- To improve on the limited efficacy of allergen avoidance.

Allergic Asthma
- In the past, the role of IT in allergic asthma had been controversial, but two large meta-analyses confirmed effectiveness of IT in treating mild-to-moderate allergic asthma compared to placebo.[14,15]
  - These studies demonstrated that patients treated with IT had reductions in allergen-specific bronchial hyperresponsiveness, medication requirements, and overall symptoms.
  - Therefore, IT has been endorsed by the WHO for the treatment of mild-to-moderate allergic asthma.[11]
- Starting IT early in the course of allergic asthma may lead to decreased use of medications and, perhaps, even an alteration in the natural course of the disease.

Insect-Sting Hypersensitivity
- Effectiveness of IT for venom hypersensitivity has been well established.
- IT is indicated for patients with a history of anaphylaxis from venom.[16]
- Patients with recurrent, large, local reactions are also candidates for venom IT.[17]

Immunotherapy Protocols
- Allergen IT needs to be individualized to the patient.
- IT is traditionally given at weekly intervals while increasing the dose to maintenance therapy.
- Rush protocols (injections given daily) and cluster protocols (multiple injections/day) are used more commonly in Europe. The exception is for insect-sting hypersensitivity, in which rush protocols are used more commonly.
- Maintenance dosages for aeroallergens are usually given every 2–4 weeks.
- Venom IT may be given every 8 weeks.
- A sample schedule for perennial aqueous IT is given in Appendix C.
- Allergen extract concentrations can be expressed as a weight per volume ratio (w/v), protein nitrogen unit (PNU), or, the biologically active measure, in allergen units (BAU).
- The goal is to attain the highest tolerated dose; usually 6–12 μg per injection of the major allergen is required.
- **A physician needs to be immediately available with proper equipment on hand in case a severe reaction occurs.**
- The recommended injection site is the outer aspect of the upper arm between the deltoid and triceps muscles.
- Extracts are administered subcutaneously.
- Oral antihistamines and leukotriene antagonists may be given to reduce local reactions.
- The patient should be **observed for at least 20–30 minutes after each injection.**[11] Life-threatening anaphylactic reactions after the initial 30 minutes are rare. Fatalities are also rare.[18]

Duration of Treatment
- Therapy is generally given for 3–5 years; however, the actual length of time for treatment is unclear.

- The recommendation of 3–5 years duration is based on data from venom hypersensitivity and only one study of a single seasonal allergen (grass); clearly, further studies need to be performed.[3]
- If symptoms are well controlled after this time, IT may be stopped.
- Some patients experience return of symptoms within 1–2 years after cessation of IT; if desired, it may be restarted but needs to be incrementally increased to the maintenance dose.
- If clinical benefit from IT is not apparent after 1–2 years, IT should be discontinued.

Side Effects and Risks

- A physician needs to be nearby to treat potentially serious reaction to IT.[11]
- **Local reactions to IT are common.**
  - Significant local reactions are identified as an immediate redness and swelling with wheal >2 cm in diameter or wheal lasting >24 hours.
  - Local reactions should be treated with oral antihistamine and local application of cold packs.
  - If significant local reaction occurs, the next dose is reduced to the previously tolerated dose.
  - Premedication with antihistamines may help reduce local reactions.
  - However, in venom IT, studies suggest that initial antihistamine premedication might actually increase the efficacy of IT.[19]
- **Systemic reactions and anaphylaxis are rare but can occur.**
  - **A fatal systemic reaction occurs in approximately one of every 2 million doses of IT administered annually.**[18,20]
  - Signs/symptoms of systemic reaction (one or more of the following): generalized erythema and/or urticaria, pruritus, angioedema, bronchospasm, laryngeal edema, and shock/cardiac arrest.
  - **Systemic/anaphylaxis reactions should be treated with IM aqueous epinephrine (0.3–0.5 mL of 1:1,000).** (see Chap. 13).
  - To limit systemic absorption of the antigen, a tourniquet should be placed above the injection site and released every 15 minutes.
  - Optionally, epinephrine 0.1–0.3 mL may also be given at the injection site to further delay absorption of the antigen.
  - Proper emergency resuscitation protocol should be followed to ensure patent airway and maintenance of adequate blood pressure.
  - Because of its more rapid onset, the preferred antihistamine is diphenhydramine and it is given IV or IM.
  - IV hydrocortisone (5 mg/kg) may be used for severe systemic reactions; however, **corticosteroids have limited effect in the immediate response.** In general, they are used to prevent a late-phase response, which may occur 4–12 hours after the initial response and can be as severe.

Relative Contraindications and Special Considerations

- **IT should not be initiated in allergic asthma patients whose asthma is unstable or poorly controlled.** The risk of fatal or near fatal events is much higher in this group.[21]
- Ongoing treatment with a β-adrenergic blocker is a relative contraindication for receiving IT. Patients receiving β-blockers are at increased risk for a severe anaphylactic reaction that may be resistant to epinephrine administration.

- Discontinuation of **angiotensin-converting enzyme (ACE) inhibitor** use should be considered before initiating venom IT due to the potential increased risk of more severe anaphylaxis.[22]
- Patients with a fever, an asthmatic with upper respiratory infection, a wheezing patient, or a patient with significantly reduced pulmonary function tests (peak expiratory flow rate [PEFR] <70% of predicted) should wait for resolution of these symptoms to receive scheduled IT.
- Strenuous exercise should be avoided immediately after an injection.
- Women who become pregnant can continue their scheduled IT at lower doses than normal. IT is not initiated in pregnant patients.
- Tryptase levels should be measured in all patients before initiating venom IT. **Higher baseline tryptase correlates with an increased risk of systemic reactions.**[23]

Potential Reasons for Failure of Immunotherapy

- Environmental modifications to control allergens are inadequate or insufficient.
- Significant or contributing allergen not recognized and omitted in IT regimen.
- Inadequate doses of major allergen in preparation (normally need 6–12 μg of the major allergen to be successful).
- New allergies develop during treatment course.
- Exposure to nonallergen triggers like cigarette smoke.
- Original causative allergen is misdiagnosed.

REFERRAL

IT should be administered by a specialist trained in allergy and immunology.

PATIENT EDUCATION

- All patients should be provided and educated in use of self-injectable epinephrine.
- Patients should be educated regarding the possible signs and symptoms of systemic reactions.
- Before IT is started, the patient should be educated about the benefits and risks of IT, as well as the methods for minimizing risks.
- Realistic outcome from IT should also be discussed with each patient.

MONITORING/FOLLOW-UP

- **Patients should be monitored for at least 20–30 minutes after receiving** IT for any adverse symptoms.
- Patients should be seen for a follow-up visit with the physician at least every 6–12 months. More frequent visits may be needed depending on response to therapy, adverse reactions, modifications in dosage or alteration in underlying allergic diseases.

OUTCOME/PROGNOSIS

- IT has been shown to significantly improve symptoms in patients with allergic rhinitis, asthma, and venom hypersensitivity.
- After 10 years, 15% of patients who underwent venom IT relapsed.[24]

REFERENCES

1. Till SJ, Francis JN, Nouri-Aria K, et al. Mechanisms of immunotherapy. *J Allergy Clin Immunol.* 2004;113:1025–1034.
2. Blaser K, Akdis CA. Interleukin-10, T regulatory cells and specific allergy treatment. *Clin Exp Allergy.* 2004;34:328–331.
3. Durham SR, Walker SM, Varga EM, et al. Long-term clinical efficacy of grass-pollen immunotherapy. *N Engl J Med.* 1999;341:468–475.
4. Lowell FC, Franklin WF, Williams M. A double-blind study of the effectiveness and specificity of injection therapy in ragweed hay fever. *N Engl J Med.* 1965;273:675–679.
5. Varney VA, Gaga M, Frew AJ, et al. Usefulness of immunotherapy in patients with severe summer hay fever uncontrolled by antiallergic drugs. *BMJ.* 1991;302:265–269.
6. Bousquet J, Demoly P, Michel FB. Specific immunotherapy in rhinitis and asthma. *Ann Allergy Asthma Immunol.* 2001;87:38–42.
7. Abramson MJ, Puy RM, Weiner JM. Injection allergen immunotherapy for asthma. *Cochrane Database Syst Rev.* 2010;(8):CD001186.
8. Eng PA, Borer-Reinhold M, Heijnen IA, et al. Twelve-year follow-up after discontinuation of preseasonal grass pollen immunotherapy in childhood. *Allergy.* 2006;61:198–201.
9. Jacobsen L, Niggemann B, Dreborg S, et al. Specific immunotherapy has long-term preventive effect of seasonal and perennial asthma: 10-year follow-up on the PAT study. *Allergy.* 2007;62:943–948.
10. Joint Task Force on Practice Parameters, American Academy of Allergy, Asthma and Immunology, American College of Allergy, Asthma and Immunology, Joint Council of Allergy, Asthma and Immunology. Allergen immunotherapy: a practice parameter second update. *J Allergy Clin Immunol.* 2007;120:S25–S85.
11. Theodoropoulos DS, Lockey RF. Allergen immunotherapy: guidelines, update, and recommendations of the World Health Organization. *Allergy Asthma Proc.* 2000;21:159–166.
12. Joint Task Force on Practice Parameters. Allergen immunotherapy: a practice parameter. American Academy of Allergy, Asthma and Immunology. American College of Allergy, Asthma and Immunology. *Ann Allergy Asthma Immunol.* 2003;90:1–40.
13. Cox L, Nelson H, Lockey R, et al. Allergen immunotherapy: a practice parameter third update. *J Allergy Clin Immunol.* 2011;127:S1–S55.
14. Abramson M, Puy R, Weiner J. Immunotherapy in asthma: an updated systematic review. *Allergy* 1999;54:1022–1041.
15. Abramson MJ, Puy RM, Weiner JM. Is allergen immunotherapy effective in asthma? A meta-analysis of randomized controlled trials. *Am J Respir Crit Care Med.* 1995;151:969–974.
16. Hunt KJ, Valentine MD, Sobotka AK, et al. A controlled trial of immunotherapy in insect hypersensitivity. *N Engl J Med.* 1978;299:157–161.
17. Golden DB, Kelly D, Hamilton RG, et al. Venom immunotherapy reduces large local reactions to insect stings. *J Allergy Clin Immunol.* 2009;123:1371–1375.
18. Lockey RF, Nicoara-Kasti GL, Theodoropoulos DS, et al. Systemic reactions and fatalities associated with allergen immunotherapy. *Ann Allergy Asthma Immunol.* 2001;87(suppl 1):47–55.
19. Muller UR. New developments in the diagnosis and treatment of hymenoptera venom allergy. *Int Arch Allergy Immunol.* 2001;124:447–453.
20. Stewart GE 2nd, Lockey RF. Systemic reactions from allergen immunotherapy. *J Allergy Clin Immunol.* 1992;90:567–578.

21. Bernstein DI, Wanner M, Borish L, et al. Twelve-year survey of fatal reactions to allergen injections and skin testing: 1990–2001. *J Allergy Clin Immunol.* 2004;113:1129–1136.
22. Moffitt JE, Golden DB, Reisman RE, et al. Stinging insect hypersensitivity: a practice parameter update. *J Allergy Clin Immunol.* 2004;114:869–886.
23. Rueff F, Przybilla B, Bilo MB, et al. Predictors of side effects during the buildup phase of venom immunotherapy for hymenoptera venom allergy: the importance of baseline serum tryptase. *J Allergy Clin Immunol.* 2010;126:105–111.
24. Golden DB, Kagey-Sobotka A, Lichtenstein LM. Survey of patients after discontinuing venom immunotherapy. *J Allergy Clin Immunol.* 2000;105:385–390.

Common Medications Used in Allergy and Immunology

TABLE A-1 ANTIHISTAMINES

Generic name	Brand name(s)	Adult dosage
First generation		
Diphenhydramine	Benadryl	25–50 q4–6h prn
Chlorpheniramine	Chlor-Trimeton, others	4 mg q4–6h prn
Brompheniramine	Dimetapp, others	4 mg q4–6h prn
Hydroxyzine	Atarax, Vistaril	25–100 mg qd–qid prn
Second generation		
Cetirizine	Zyrtec	5 or 10 mg qd
Levocetirizine	Xyzal	2.5 or 5 mg qd
Fexofenadine	Allegra	60 mg bid or 180 mg qd
Loratadine	Claritin	10 mg qd
Desloratadine	Clarinex	5 mg qd

TABLE A-2 INTRANASAL CORTICOSTEROIDS

Generic name	Brand name(s)	Adult dosage
Beclomethasone dipropionate	Beconase AQ	42 μg/spray: 1–2 sprays each nostril bid
	Vancenase AQ	84 μg/spray: 1–2 sprays each nostril qd
Budesonide	Rhinocort Aqua	32 μg/spray: 1–4 sprays each nostril qd
Flunisolide	Nasalide, Nasarel	25 μg/spray: 2 sprays each nostril bid
Fluticasone propionate	Flonase	50 μg/spray: 2 sprays each nostril qd or 1 spray each nostril bid
Fluticasone furoate	Veramyst, Avamys	27.5 μg/spray: 2 sprays each nostril qd
Mometasone furoate	Nasonex	50 μg/spray: 2 sprays each nostril qd
Ciclesonide	Omnaris	50 μg/spray: 2 sprays each nostril qd
Triamcinolone acetonide	Nasacort AQ	55 μg/spray: 2 sprays each nostril qd

TABLE A-3	INTRANASAL ANTIHISTAMINES	
Generic name	Brand name(s)	Adult dosage
Olopatadine	Patanase	665 µg/spray: 2 sprays each nostril bid
Azelastine	Astelin	137 µg/spray: 2 sprays each nostril bid
	Astepro	205.5 µg/spray: 2 sprays each nostril bid

TABLE A-4	OTHER INTRANASAL PREPARATIONS	
Ipratropium bromide	Atrovent	0.03% (21 µg/spray): 2 sprays each nostril bid–tid
		0.06% (42 µg/spray): 2 sprays each nostril tid–qid

TABLE A-5	OPHTHALMIC ANTIALLERGY PREPARATIONS	
Generic name	Brand name(s)	Adult dosage
Antihistamines/decongestants		
Naphazoline + pheniramine	Naphcon-A, Opcon-A, Visine-A	1 drop qid prn
Naphazoline + antazoline	Vasocon-A	1 drop qid prn
Antihistamines		
Levocabastine 0.05%	Livostin	1 drop qid prn
Emedastine 0.05%	Emadine	1 drop qid prn
Epinastine 0.05%	Elestat	1 drop bid
Azelastine 0.05%	Optivar	1 drop bid
Antihistamines/mast cell stabilizer		
Olopatadine 0.1%	Patanol	1 drop bid
Olopatadine 0.2%	Pataday	1 drop qd
Ketotifen fumarate 0.025%	Zaditor	1 drop q8–12h
Mast cell stabilizers		
Lodoxamide tromethamine 0.1%	Alomide	1 drop qid
Nedocromil sodium 2%	Alocril	1 drop bid
Cromolyn sodium 4%	Crolom, Opticrom	1 drop q4–6h
Pemirolast potassium 0.1%	Alamast	1 drop qid
Nonsteroidal anti-inflammatory drugs		
Ketorolac tromethamine 0.4%	Acular LS	1 drop qid
Diclofenac sodium 0.1%	Voltaren Ophthalmic	1 drop qid
Steroids		
Prednisolone acetate 0.12%	Pred Mild	1 drop bid–qid
Loteprednol etabonate 0.2%	Alrex	1 drop qid
Loteprednol etabonate 0.5%	Lotemax	1 drop qid

TABLE A-6 INHALED β_2-AGONISTS

Generic name	Brand name(s)	Adult dosage
Short acting		
Albuterol sulfate	Proventil, Ventolin, ProAir	Nebulized (5 mg/mL): 2.5 mg q6–8h prn MDI (90 μg/puff): 2 puffs q4–6h prn
Levalbuterol	Xopenex	Nebulized: 0.63–1.25 mg tid prn MDI (45 μg/puff): 2 puffs q4–6h prn
Pirbuterol acetate	Maxair, Maxair Autohaler	MDI or Autohaler (200 μg/puff): 2 puffs q4–6h prn
Long acting[a]		
Salmeterol	Serevent Diskus	Dry-powder inhaler (50 μg/inhalation): 1 inhalation q12h
Formoterol fumarate	Foradil Aerolizer	Dry-powder inhaler (12 μg/inhalation): 1 inhalation q12h

[a]Long-acting β-agonists should not be used as monotherapy for asthma and should be co-administered with inhaled corticosteroids (Chapter 4).

TABLE A-7 INHALED CORTICOSTEROIDS

Generic name	Brand name(s)	Preparations	Adult dose	Adult equivalent dosage[a]		
				Low dose (μg/day)	Medium dose (μg/day)	High dose (μg/day)
Beclomethasone dipropionate	QVAR	MDI: 40 or 80 μg/inhalation	40–160 μg BID	80–240	>240–480	>480
Budesonide	Pulmicort Flexhaler	Dry-powder inhaler: 90 or 180 μg/inhalation		180–600	>600–1200	>1200
Mometasone	Asmanex Twisthaler[c]	Dry-powder inhaler: 220 μg/inhalation		220	440	>440
Fluticasone proprionate	Flovent	MDI: 44, 110, 220 μg/puff Dry-powder inhaler: 50, 100, 250 μg/inhalation		88–264	>264–440	>440
Ciclesonide	Alvesco	MDI: 80, 160 μg/puff		100–300 [b]	>300–500 [b]	>500 [b]

[a]Summary Report 2007. National Institutes of Health. National Heart, Lung, and Blood Institute. National Asthma Education and Prevention Program Expert Panel Report 3 (EPR-3): Guidelines for the Diagnosis and Management of Asthma. NIH Publication 08-5846. Bethesda, MD, August 2007.

[b]Estimated comparative dose not available from above. Recommended dose is 80–320 μg bid.

[c]Approved for once daily dosing.

TABLE A-8 LEUKOTRIENE MODIFIERS

Generic name	Brand name	Adult dosage
Montelukast	Singulair	10 mg qhs
Zafirlukast	Accolate	20 mg bid
Zileuton	Zyflo	600 mg qid
	Zyflo CR	1200 mg bid

TABLE A-9 OTHER ASTHMA DRUGS

Generic name	Brand name(s)	Adult dosage
Mast cell stabilizers		
Cromolyn sodium		Nebulizer solution (20 mg/ ampule): 1 ampule qid
Xanthine derivatives		
Theophylline	Uniphyl, Theo-24, Exiophyllin, various	300–600 mg/day
Combined inhaled corticosteroid and long-acting β-agonist		
Mometasone + formoterol	Dulera	MDI (100/200 μg mometasone + 5 μg formoterol/inhalation): 2 puffs bid
Budesonide + formoterol	Symbicort	MDI (80/160 μg budesonide + 4.5 μg formoterol/inhalation): 2 puffs bid
Fluticasone + salmeterol	Advair HFA	HFA (45/115/230 μg fluticasone + 21 μg salmeterol/inhalation): 2 puffs bid
	Advair Diskus	Dry-inhalation powder (100/250/500 μg fluticasone + 50 μg salmeterol/inhalation): 1 inhalation bid

TABLE A-10   SELECTED TOPICAL CORTICOSTEROIDS

Generic name	Brand name(s)	Vehicle
Very high potency		
Betamethasone dipropionate, augmented 0.05%	Diprolene	Ointment
Clobetasol propionate 0.05%	Temovate, others	Cream, ointment, gel
Halobetasol propionate 0.05%	Ultravate	Cream, ointment
High potency		
Amcinonide 0.1%	Cyclocort	Cream, ointment, lotion
Betamethasone dipropionate, augmented 0.05%	Diprolene AF	Cream
Betamethasone dipropionate 0.05%	Diprosone, others	Cream, ointment
Betamethasone valerate 0.1%	Betatrex	Ointment
Desoximetasone 0.05%	Topicort	Gel
Desoximetasone 0.25%	Topicort	Cream, ointment
Fluocinonide 0.05%	Lidex, others	Cream, ointment, gel
Halcinonide 0.1%	Halog, Halog-E	Cream, ointment
Triamcinolone acetonide 0.5%	Aristocort, Kenalog, others	Cream, ointment, lotion
Intermediate potency		
Betamethasone dipropionate 0.05%	Diprosone, others	Lotion
Betamethasone valerate 0.1%	Betatrex, Valisone	Cream, lotion
Desoximetasone 0.05%, 0.25%	Topicort	Cream, ointment, gel
Fluocinolone acetonide 0.025%	Synalar	Cream, ointment
Flurandrenolide 0.025%, 0.05%	Cordran	Cream, ointment, lotion
Fluticasone propionate 0.005%	Cutivate	Ointment
Fluticasone propionate 0.05%	Cutivate	Cream
Hydrocortisone butyrate 0.1%	Locoid	Cream, ointment, solution
Hydrocortisone valerate 0.2%	Westcort	Cream, ointment
Mometasone furoate 0.1%	Elocon	Cream, ointment, lotion
Triamcinolone acetonide 0.025%, 0.1%	Aristocort, Kenalog, others	Cream, ointment, lotion
Low potency		
Alclometasone dipropionate 0.05%	Aclovate	Cream, ointment
Desonide 0.05%	DesOwen	Cream, lotion, ointment
Dexamethasone sodium phosphate 0.1%	Decadron	Cream, gel
Fluocinolone acetonide 0.01%	Synalar	Cream, ointment
Hydrocortisone acetate 0.5%, 1%	Cortaid, others	Cream, ointment
Hydrocortisone 1%, 2.5%	Hytone, others	Cream, ointment, lotion

Note: Adult dosages range from qd to qid (consult labels).

TABLE A-11 GLUCOCORTICOID EQUIVALENCIES, POTENCIES, AND HALF-LIVES

Glucocorticoid	Approximate equivalent dose (mg)	Relative anti-inflammatory (glucocorticoid) potency	Relative mineralocorticoid potency	Pregnancy category	Half-life	
					Plasma (minutes)	Biologic (hours)
Short-acting						
Cortisone	25	0.8	2	D	30	8–12
Hydrocortisone	20	1	2	C	80–118	8–12
Intermediate-acting						
Prednisone	5	4	1	B	60	18–36
Prednisolone	5	4	1	B	115–212	18–36
Triamcinolone	4	5	0	C	200+	18–36
Methylprednisolone	4	5	0	C	78–188	18–36
Long-acting						
Dexamethasone	0.75	20–30	0	C	110–210	36–54
Betamethasone	0.6–0.75	25	0	C	300+	36–54

TABLE A-12	ANAPHYLAXIS KITS	
Generic name	Brand name	Adult dosage
Epinephrine (1:1,000; 1 mg/mL)	EpiPen	Auto-injector (0.30 mg): 1 injection IM (0.30 mg injector recommended for most adults)
	Twinject	Epinephrine auto-injector containing two 0.30 mg doses: 1 injection IM, repeat if needed in 5–15 minutes

Lab Values for Selected Tests in Immunology

TABLE B-1 COMPLETE BLOOD COUNT—ADULT		
Normal range	**Adult male**	**Adult female**
White blood cells (k/m^3)	3.8–9.8	3.8–9.8
Red blood cells (m/m^3)	4.5–5.7	3.9–5
Hemoglobin (g/dL)	13.8–17.2	12.1–15.1
Hematocrit (%)	40.7–50.3	36.1–44.3
Platelets (k/m^3)	140–440	140–440

TABLE B-2 WHITE BLOOD CELL COUNT AND DIFFERENTIAL—CHILDREN

Age	WBC (× 10^3/mm³)	Segs	Bands	Lymphs	Monos	Eosinophils	Basophils	Atypical lymphs	NRBCs
0–3 days	9.0–35.0	32–62	10–18	19–29	5–7	0–2	0–1	0–8	0–2
1–2 weeks	5.0–20.0	14–34	6–14	36–45	6–10	0–2	0–1	0–8	0
1–6 months	6.0–17.5	13–33	4–12	41–71	4–7	0–3	0–1	0–8	0
7 months to 2 years	6.0–17.0	15–35	5–11	45–76	3–6	0–3	0–1	0–8	0
2–5 years	5.5–15.5	23–45	5–11	35–65	3–6	0–3	0–1	0–8	0
5–8 years	5.0–14.5	32–54	5–11	28–48	3–6	0–3	0–1	0–8	0
13–18 years	4.5–13.0	34–64	5–11	25–45	3–6	0–3	0–1	0–8	0

Lymphs, lymphocytes; monos, monocytes; NRBC, nucleated red blood cells; segs, segmented neutrophils.

With permission American Academy of Pediatrics, https://www.pediatriccareonline.org/pco/ub/view/Pediatric-Drug-Lookup/153930/0/normal_laboratory_values_for_children?amod = aapea&login = true&nfstatus = 401&nftoken = 00000000-0000-0000-0000-000000000000&nfstatusdescription = ERROR%3a+No+local+token. Last accessed: December 7, 2011.

TABLE B-3	QUANTITATIVE IMMUNOGLOBULIN RANGE BY AGE		
Reference ranges	IgG (mg/dL)	IgA (mg/dL)	IgM (mg/dL)
Cord blood	636–1,660	1.4–3.8	6.3–25
1–12 months	251–1,069	2.9–125	20–149
1–4 years	345–1,213	14–159	43–200
5–8 years	463–1,280	25–202	48–207
9 years to adult	608–1,572	45–312	52–352
Adult	700–1,450	70–370	30–210

TABLE B-4	FLOW CYTOMETRY FOR CD4/CD3/CD8—IMMUNE COMPETENCE PANEL, ADULTS	
	Normal range (%)	Absolute numbers
CD3 (T cell)	54–87	650–1,770
CD4 (helper T cell)	32–60	400–1,175
CD8 (cytotoxic T cell)	13–43	145–820
CD19 (B cell)	18–25	1,000–2,200

TABLE B-5	VACCINATION RESPONSE

Haemophilus influenzae type B antibody >1.0 μ/mL	Used to test protein antigen-specific responses in immunized individuals
Tetanus >0.1 units/mL	Used to test protein antigen responses in immunized individuals
Streptococus pneumoniae Serotype specific IgG: 1.3 μg/mL in >50% response in children and >70% in adults	Used to test polysaccharide antigen responses in immunized individuals

TABLE B-6	LYMPHOCYTE MITOGEN STUDIES

Phytohemagglutinin	47,318–229,629 cpm T-cell mitogen
Pokeweed mitogen	14,087–86,429 cpm T-cell dependent B-cell mitogen
Concanavalin A	35,275–176,670 cpm T-cell mitogen

Note: These tests are performed by measuring incorporation of tritiated thymidine into lymphocytes stimulated with mitogens listed. Counts per minute (cpm) indicates amount of thymidine incorporation. Unstimulated lymphocytes incorporate <1,000 cpm. Values are usually expressed as a percentage compared to normal healthy control.

TABLE B-7 CELL-SUBSET COUNTS OF PERIPHERAL BLOOD LYMPHOCYTES IN HEALTHY CHILDREN

Subset	N	0–3 months	3–6 months	6–12 months	1–2 years	2–6 years	6–12 years	12–18 years
WBC	800	10.60 (7.20–18.00)	9.20 (6.70–14.00)	9.10 (6.40–13.00)	8.80 (6.40–12.00)	7.10 (5.20–11.00)	6.50 (4.40–9.50)	6.00 (4.40–8.10)
Lymphocyte	800	5.40 (3.40–7.60)	6.30 (3.90–9.00)	5.90 (3.40–9.00)	5.50 (3.60–8.90)	3.60 (2.30–5.40)	2.70 (1.90–3.70)	2.20 (1.40–3.30)
3	699	3.68 (2.50–5.50)	3.93 (2.50–5.60)	3.93 (1.90–5.90)	3.55 (2.10–6.20)	2.39 (1.40–3.70)	1.82 (1.20–2.60)	1.48 (1.00–2.20)
19	699	0.73 (0.30–2.00)	1.55 (0.43–3.00)	1.52 (0.61–2.60)	1.31 (0.72–2.60)	0.75 (0.39–1.40)	0.48 (0.27–0.86)	0.30 (0.11–0.57)
16/56	770	0.42 (0.17–1.10)	0.42 (0.17–0.83)	0.40 (0.16–0.95)	0.36 (0.18–0.92)	0.30 (0.13–0.72)	0.23 (0.10–0.48)	0.19 (0.07–0.48)
4	699	2.61 (1.60–4.00)	2.85 (1.80–4.00)	2.67 (1.40–4.30)	2.16 (1.30–3.40)	1.38 (0.70–2.20)	0.98 (0.65–1.50)	0.84 (0.53–1.30)
8	699	0.98 (0.56–1.70)	1.05 (0.59–1.60)	1.04 (0.50–1.70)	1.04 (0.62–2.00)	0.84 (0.49–1.30)	0.68 (0.37–1.10)	0.53 (0.33–0.92)
4/45RA/62L	694	2.25 (1.20–3.60)	2.23 (1.30–3.60)	2.10 (1.10–3.60)	1.64 (0.95–2.80)	0.96 (0.42–1.50)	0.56 (0.31–1.00)	0.39 (0.21–0.75)
8/45RA/62L	696	0.73 (0.38–1.30)	0.74 (0.45–1.20)	0.70 (0.33–1.20)	0.76 (0.40–1.40)	0.54 (0.26–0.85)	0.41 (0.20–0.65)	0.30 (0.17–0.56)
4/45RA	694	2.27 (1.20–3.70)	2.32 (1.30–3.70)	2.21 (1.10–3.70)	1.65 (1.00–2.90)	0.98 (0.43–1.50)	0.57 (0.32–1.00)	0.40 (0.23–0.77)
8/45RA	696	0.87 (0.45–1.50)	0.91 (0.55–1.40)	0.87 (0.48–1.50)	0.94 (0.49–1.70)	0.67 (0.38–1.10)	0.54 (0.31–0.90)	0.40 (0.24–0.71)
4/DR/38	694	0.08 (0.03–0.18)	0.11 (0.05–0.26)	0.10 (0.04–0.22)	0.10 (0.05–0.25)	0.06 (0.03–0.14)	0.04 (0.02–0.08)	0.03 (0.01–0.06)
8/DR/38	697	0.05 (0.02–0.16)	0.07 (0.03–0.17)	0.09 (0.04–0.27)	0.18 (0.05–0.54)	0.11 (0.05–0.34)	0.06 (0.03–0.18)	0.04 (0.02–0.13)

	N							
4/DR	694	0.10 (0.04–0.18)	0.15 (0.06–028)	0.12 (0.05–0.26)	0.13 (0.07–0.28)	0.09 (0.05–0.18)	0.07 (0.04–0.12)	0.06 (0.03–0.10)
8/DR	697	0.05 (0.02–0.16)	0.08 (0.03–0.17)	0.09 (0.04–0.29)	0.18 (0.06–0.60)	0.14 (0.07–0.42)	0.09 (0.04–0.27)	0.07 (0.03–0.18)
4/38	694	2.54 (0.16–3.90)	2.77 (1.60–4.00)	2.55 (1.20–4.10)	2.02 (1.20–3.30)	1.21 (0.59–2.00)	0.75 (0.48–1.20)	0.57 (0.33–1.00)
8/38	697	0.93 (0.55–1.60)	0.94 (0.53–1.50)	0.93 (0.45–1.60)	0.95 (0.57–1.90)	0.67 (0.39–1.10)	0.48 (0.24–0.74)	0.31 (0.16–5.70)
4/28	695	2.56 (1.60–3.80)	2.65 (1.60–4.00)	2.58 (1.20–4.20)	2.12 (1.30–3.40)	1.33 (0.69–2.00)	0.94 (0.63–1.50)	0.79 (0.49–1.20)
8/28	696	0.71 (0.35–1.30)	0.73 (0.35–1.20)	0.67 (0.28–1.10)	0.72 (0.40–1.30)	0.50 (0.28–0.87)	0.40 (0.21–0.70)	0.29 (0.16–0.52)
4/95	695	0.29 (0.16–0.58)	0.41 (0.23–0.62)	0.51 (0.29–0.82)	0.50 (0.27–0.91)	0.42 (0.27–0.65)	0.36 (0.25–0.62)	0.40 (0.25–0.66)
8/95	696	0.12 (0.05–0.31)	0.16 (0.06–0.39)	0.22 (0.08–0.66)	0.34 (0.10–0.85)	0.30 (0.11–0.58)	0.25 (0.08–0.53)	0.21 (0.08–0.45)
3/4/45RO	644	0.32 (0.06–0.90)	0.33 (0.12–0.63)	0.34 (0.16–0.80)	0.40 (0.21–0.85)	0.36 (0.22–0.66)	0.35 (0.23–0.63)	0.38 (0.24–0.70)
3/4-/45RO	644	0.10 (0.03–0.33)	0.12 (0.03–0.29)	0.12 (0.04–0.33)	0.23 (0.06–0.57)	0.19 (0.09–0.44)	0.21 (0.07–0.39)	0.16 (0.06–0.31)
3/45RO	644	0.48 (0.09–1.20)	0.46 (0.15–086)	0.47 (0.22–1.10)	0.65 (0.30–1.30)	0.57 (0.33–1.00)	0.59 (0.32–0.95)	0.56 (0.34–0.97)
3/19/38	655	0.60 (0.12–2.00)	1.20 (0.00–2.80)	1.29 (0.02–2.20)	1.04 (0.00–2.20)	0.56 (0.01–1.20)	0.28 (0.00–0.67)	0.03 (0.00–0.35)
3/19	655	0.62 (0.12–2.10)	1.26 (0.00–2.80)	1.33 (0.02–2.30)	1.10 (0.00–2.30)	0.67 (0.02–1.40)	0.34 (0.00–0.74)	0.04 (0.00–0.39)

With permission Shearer WT, Rosenblatt HM, Gelman RS, et al. Lymphocyte subsets in healthy children from birth through 18 years of age: the Pediatric AIDS Clinical Trials Group P1009 study. J Allergy Clin Immunol. 2003;112:973–980.

Sample Schedule for Perennial Aqueous Immunotherapy

SAMPLE BUILDUP FOR WEEKLY IMMUNOTHERAPY AND SUGGESTED METHODS FOR LABELING DILUTIONS

Dilution	Volume (mL)
1:1,000	0.05
Number 4 or green	0.1
	0.3
	0.5
1:100	0.05
Number 3 or blue	0.1
	0.2
	0.3
	0.4
	0.5
1:10	0.05
Number 2 or yellow	0.05
	0.1
	0.2
	0.3
	0.35
	0.4
	0.45
	0.5
1:1 Maintenance concentrate	0.05
Number 1 or red	0.1
	0.15
	0.2
	0.25
	0.3
	0.35
	0.4
	0.45
	0.5

Note: Dilutions expressed as volume/volume from the maintenance concentrate vaccine.

Reprinted with permission from: Joint Task Force on Practice Parameters. Allergen immunotherapy: a practice parameter. American Academy of Allergy, Asthma and Immunology. American College of Allergy, Asthma and Immunology. *Ann Allergy Asthma Imunol.* 2003;90:1–40.

Index

Note: Page locators followed by f and t indicates figure and table respectively.

A

Acute bacterial rhinosinusitis, 18
  symptoms of, 18
  treatment of, 20
Acute contact dermatitis, 128
Acute eosinophilic pneumonia (AEP), 144, 148
  treatment of, 151
Acute interstitial nephritis (AIN), 107–108
Acute lymphoblastic leukemia (ALL), 143
Acute myeloid leukemia (AML), 143
Acute rhinosinusitis (ARS), 17
Acute sinusitis, 17
Adaptive immune system, 4
  CD4+ T cells, 4
  cellular immunity, 4
  humoral immunity, 4
Adverse drug reaction (ADR), 103.
    See also Drug allergy
  classification of, 103
  definition of, 103
  epidemiology of, 103
  predictable adverse reactions, 103
  unpredictable adverse reactions, 103
Adverse food reaction, 125
Aeroallergen skin testing
  for asthma, 30
Aggressive systemic mastocytosis (ASM), 156
Airway inflammation and
    bronchoconstriction, 26
Airway management, for anaphylaxis, 101
Airway obstruction, in pulmonary function
    tests, 54
Allergen immunotherapy (IT), 173–179.
    See also Immunotherapy, allergen
Allergens, 4, 5, 9
  T.R.U.E. test panel of, 66t
Allergic bronchopulmonary aspergillosis
    (ABPA), 33, 140
Allergic contact dermatitis (ACD), 85–88.
    See also Dermatitis
  diagnostic testing for, 64–65
Allergic contact urticaria, 136
Allergic drug reactions, clinical criteria of,
    108t
Allergic fungal sinusitis, 19

Allergic patient
  diagnosis of
    environmental history, 1
    family history of, 2
    food allergy history, 2
    general appearance, 2
    head and neck, 2
    history of, 1
    pulmonary, 2
    pulmonary testing, 3
    skin, 2–3
    skin testing, 3
    in vitro tests, 3
Allergic response
  immediate response, 6
  late-phase reaction, 6
Allergic rhinitis (AR)
  causes of, 8, 9
  characteristics of, 8
  classification of, 8–9
  complications of, 15
  definition of, 8
  diagnosis of
    clinical presentation of, 10–11
    diagnostic testing, 12–13
    differential diagnosis of, 11–12, 11t
  elderly patients and, 15
  epidemiology of, 9
  episodic, 9
  etiology of, 9
  monitoring of, 16
  nonpharmacologic therapies, 14–15
  pathophysiology of, 9
  perennial, 9
  and pregnancy, 15
  referral of, 15–16, 16t
  risk factors of, 9–10
  seasonal, 8
  symptoms of, 8
  treatment of, 13–14
Allergic salute, 2, 11
Allergic shiners, 2, 11
Allergy, 4. *See also* specific allergies
  basic immunology of, 4–7
  classification of, 5
  definition of, 1

Allergy (*Continued*)
  etiology of, 5–7
  initial diagnosis of
    history in, 1–2
    physical examination in, 2–3
    skin testing in, 3
    in vivo and *in vitro* diagnostic tests of
      diagnosis of, 59–66, 62t, 64t
      principles of, 59
Alveolitis, extrinsic allergic. *See*
      Pneumonitis, hypersensitivity
The American Academy of Allergy, Asthma,
      and Immunology (AAAAI), 18
American Academy of Otolaryngology-
      Head and Neck Surgery, 18
American College of Physicians', 18
American Latex Allergy Association, 138
American Thoracic Society, 53
Amoxicillin allergy, 112
Anaphylactoid reactions, 103
Anaphylaxis, 136
  causes of, 96
  clinical presentation of, 97–98, 98t
  definition of, 96
  diagnosis of, 97–99
  differential diagnosis of, 99t
  in drug allergy, 106
  epidemiology of, 96
  etiology of, 96
  exercise-induced, 130
  in food allergy, 125
  idiopathic, 98
  kits, 188t
  management of, 100f
  pathophysiology of, 96–97
  protracted, 98
  risk factors for, 97
  treatment of, 99–102
Anesthetics, local, allergy to
  classification of, 113–114, 114t
Angioedema, 3, 68, 128
  acquired, 69, 70
  characteristics of, 71
  classification of, 68
  definition of, 68
  diagnosis of, 70–74
  differential diagnosis of, 73
  in drug allergy, 104
  epidemiology of, 68–69
  familial syndromes of, 71
  hereditary, 70, 71
  occurrence of, 69
  pathophysiology of, 69–70
  pressure, 72
  principles of, 68
  treatment of, 74–75

Angiotensin-converting enzyme (ACE), 10,
      69, 119, 178
Antiallergy preparations, ophthalmic, 182t
Antibiotics
  for asthma, 32
  for sinusitis, 20–21
Anticholinergics, 31
Antigens, 5
Antihistamines, 181t
  for allergic rhinitis, 13
  in anaphylaxis treatment, 101
  for atopic dermatitis, 82
  intranasal, 182t
Anti-IgE therapy, 32
Antineutrophil cytoplasmic antibody
      (ANCA), 147
Antinuclear antibodies (ANA), 73
Arachidonic acid (AA), 7, 89
Arterial blood gas measurement, 30
Aspergillus fumigatus, 19, 35
Asthma, 23–35
  acute exacerbations of, 33t
  aspirin-sensitive, 26, 32
  classification of, 23, 24t–25t
  complications of, 32–35
  cough-variant, 28
  definition of, 23
  diagnosis of, 28–30
  differential diagnosis of, 29, 29t
  epidemiology of
    adult vs pediatric prevalence in, 27
    socioeconomic factors in, 26
  exercise-induced, 32
  irritant-induced (*See* Asthma,
      occupational)
  management of, 32, 34f
  mortality, 26
  natural history of, 28
  neutrophilic, 26
  non-IgE-mediated inflammation in, 26
  occupational, 37–42
    agents associated with, 38t
    causes of, 37
    classification of, 37
    diagnosis of, 39–42, 41f
    differential diagnosis of, 40
    epidemiology of, 37
    pathophysiology of, 37–39
    prevention of, 39
    risk factors for, 39
    treatment of, 42
  passive tobacco smoke exposure, 27
  pathophysiology of, 26–27
  predictive index, 27
  during pregnancy, 35
  prevention of, 27

respiratory infections, 27
risk factors of, 27
socioeconomic considerations, 26
treatment of, 30–32
Asthma drugs, 185t
Atopic dermatitis (AD), 3, 77–83, 128. *See also* Dermatitis
Atopic keratoconjunctivitis (AKC), 83, 89, 94
physical examination of, 91
risk factors for, 90
Atopic march, 28
α-Tryptase, 6
Autoimmunity, 4
Azathioprine, 81
Aztreonam, 112

B
Bacterial conjunctivitis, 92
Basophils, 7
Blood gas, in asthma management, 30
Bronchial hyperresponsiveness (BHR), 56
Bronchiolitis obliterans, 40
Bronchoalveolar lavage (BAL), 47, 148
in hypersensitivity pneumonitis diagnosis, 49
Bronchocentric granulomatosis, 146
Bronchoconstriction, 26
Bronchodilators, in anaphylaxis treatment, 101
Bronchoprovocation testing, 57t
Bronchopulmonary aspergillosis, allergic, 33, 35
β-Tryptase, 6
Budesonide, 35
Bullous pemphigoid, 73
Bumblebees, 116

C
Calcineurin inhibitors, 81
Carbapenems, 112
CD4+ T cells, 4
types of, 4
Cell-mediated immunity, 4
Cellular immunity, 4
Cephalosporins, 112
Cerebrospinal fluid (CSF), 12
Cetirizine, 15
Chest radiograph (CXR), 30
in asthma management, 30
Chlamydial conjunctivitis, 92
Chronic eosinophilic pneumonia, 144
treatment of, 151
Chronic idiopathic urticaria (CIU), 69
Chronic myelogenous leukemia (CML), 143

Chronic obstructive pulmonary disease (COPD), 30, 54
Chronic rhinosinusitis (CRS), 17
treatment of, 21
Churg–Strauss syndrome, 145, 148
treatment of, 151
Ciliary function testing, in sinusitis diagnosis, 20
Cladribine, 158
Clostridium difficile, 21
Cobblestoning, 11
Combined immunodeficiencies (CIDs), 160
Complete blood count (CBC), 19, 73, 164
of adult, 189t
Complete metabolic profile (CMP), 75
Conjunctivitis, 11
allergic, 89
bacterial, 92
chlamydial, 92
giant papillary, 89
vernal, 89
viral, 92
Contact dermatitis, 85
allergic, 136
irritant, 136
Contact urticaria, 128
Corticosteroids, 81
topical, 186t
C-reactive protein (CRP), 48
Cromolyn sodium, in asthma management, 32
Curschmann's spirals, 28
Cushing's syndrome, 29
Cutaneous mastocytosis (CM), 154
Cyclosporine, 75
Cystic fibrosis transmembrane regulator (CFTR), 164
Cytology, nasal, in sinusitis diagnosis, 20
Cytomegalovirus (CMV), 142

D
Decongestants, nasal
for allergic rhinitis, 14
in sinusitis treatment, 21
Delayed-type hypersensitivity (DTH), 165
Dennie–Morgan lines, 2
Dennie's lines, 11
Dermatitis
allergic contact
causes of, 85
classification of, 85
definition of, 85
diagnosis of, 86–87
differential diagnosis of, 87

Dermatitis (*Continued*)
  epidemiology of, 85
  history of, 86
  patch testing, 87
  pathophysiology of, 85–86
  physical examination for, 86–87
  risk factors for, 86
  sensitization phase, 85
  treatment of, 87–88
  atopic
    complications of, 83
    definition of, 77
    diagnosis of, 79–80
    dietary restriction in, 82
    differential diagnosis of, 80
    environmental and trigger control in, 82
    epidemiology of, 77
    etiology of, 77–78
    immunotherapy in, 81–82
    increased IgE in, 78
    inflammation in, 78
    medications for, 81
    natural history of, 79
    pathophysiology of, 78–79
    physical examination in, 79
    principles of, 77
    skin care and hydration in, 82–83
    specific allergens in, 82
    treatment of, 81–83
    wet-wrap dressings, 83
    workup for, 83
Dermatitis herpetiformis, 73
Dermatographism, 3
Desensitization
  for penicillin allergy, 111–112, 112t
  for prevention of drug allergy, 109
Diesel fuel exhaust particles and asthma
    risk, 26. *See also* Asthma
Diffuse cutaneous mastocytosis (DCM), 155
Diffusion capacity of carbon monoxide
    (DLCO), 47
DiGeorge syndrome, 163, 165
Dihydrorhodamine (DHR), 165
Diphenhydramine, 101, 132
Doxepin, 74
Drug allergy. *See also specific drugs*
  classification of, 103
  definition of, 103
  diagnosis of, 105–110
  diagnostic testing for, 109–110
    patch testing, 109
    skin testing, 109
    in vitro studies, 109–110
  epidemiology of, 103

graded dose challenge, 109
pathophysiology of, 103–104
  complete antigens in, 104
  haptens in, 104
  immunologic mechanisms in, 104
physical exam of
  acute interstitial nephritis in, 107–108
  anaphylaxis in, 106
  angioedema in, 106
  contact dermatitis in, 106
  drug fever in, 106
  drug-induced hepatitis in, 107
  erythema multiforme in, 107
  fixed drug reaction in, 106
  hematologic manifestations in, 108
  hemolytic anemia, 108
  maculopapular or morbilliform skin
    eruptions in, 106
  neutropenia, 108
  serum sickness syndrome in, 106
  Stevens-Johnson syndrome in, 107
  systemic lupus erythematosus, 107
  thrombocytopenia, 108
  toxic epidermal necrolysis in, 107
  urticaria in, 106
prevention of, 105
risk factors for, 104–105
treatment of, 110
Drug fever, in drug allergy, 106
Drug-induced lupus (DIL), 104
Drug-induced rhinitis, 12
Drug rash, eosinophilia, and systemic
    symptoms (DRESS), 142
Dual energy x-ray absorptiometry (DEXA),
    157

E
Ecallantide, 75
Emphysema, 54
Enzyme-linked immunosorbent assay
    (ELISA), 48
Eosinophilia
  classification of, 140
    cutaneous lesions with, 145
    parasitic infection with, 141
    pulmonary infiltrates with, 145
  definition of, 140
  dermatologic disorders, 143–144
  diagnosis of, 141–150
  differential diagnosis of, 141–147
  and gastrointestinal disorders, 146
  hematologic and neoplastic disorders,
    142–143
  history of, 141
  infectious causes, 142

medication-induced causes, 141–142
pathophysiology of, 140–141
pulmonary disorders, 144–146, 144t, 149t
treatment of, 150–152
urinary tract disorders, 146–147
Eosinophilia-myalgia syndrome, 142
Eosinophilic cellulitis, 144
Eosinophilic colitis, 146, 150
treatment of, 152
Eosinophilic cystitis, 147, 150
Eosinophilic esophagitis (EE), 125, 146, 150
treatment of, 152
Eosinophilic fasciitis, 144
Eosinophilic gastroenteritis, 146, 150
treatment of, 152
Eosinophilic granuloma, pulmonary, 145–146
Eosinophilic panniculitis, 143
Eosinophils, 7, 140
Eosinophiluria, 146
Epicutaneous skin tests, 3
for allergy, 60
prick skin testing, 60
puncture skin testing, 60
Epidermal necrolysis, toxic, 107
Epinephrine
in anaphylaxis treatment, 100
for food allergy treatment, 132
Epstein–Barr viral infection, 105
Erythema multiforme, 107. See also Drug allergy
in drug allergy, 107
minor, 73
Erythrocyte sedimentation rate (ESR), 48, 73, 147
Extrinsic allergic alveolitis. See Hypersensitivity pneumonitis (HP)
Eyelids, atopic contact dermatitis of, 94

F
FcεRI, 6
high-affinity, 6
FcεRII, 6
Filaggrin, 77
Fire ants, 116
Flexible rhinoscopy, 2
Flow cytometry
for CD4/CD3/CD8, 191t
Fluorescence in situ hybridization (FISH), 148
Food allergy (FA), 126t–127t
adjunctive treatment of, 132
classification of, 125, 128

clinical presentation of
IgE-mediated immune reactions in, 125
non–IgE-mediated immune reactions in, 125
nonimmunologic reactions in, 125
diagnosis of, 130–132
differential diagnosis of, 130
discharge therapy of, 132
epidemiology of, 128–129
IgE-mediated, 125
monitoring, 134
non-IgE-mediated, 125
pathophysiology of, 129
patient education, 133–134
prevention of, 129
risk factors for, 129
treatment of, 132–133
workup for
diet elimination in, 132
food challenges in, 131
RAST testing in, 131
skin tests in, 131
Food hypersensitivity. See Food allergy (FA)
Food-induced anaphylaxis, 125
Food intolerances, 125
Food protein–induced enterocolitis syndrome (FPIES), 128
Forced expiratory flow (FEF), 54
Forced expiratory volume at 1 second to forced vital capacity (FEV$_1$/FVC), 148
Forced vital capacity (FVC), 52
Functional residual capacity (FRC), 52

G
Gastrointestinal (GI)
disorders, 140
food allergies, 125
dietary protein–induced proctitis, 125
EoE, 125
eosinophilic gastroenteritis, 125
FPIES, 128
immediate GI hypersensitivity, 125
OAS, 128
Giant papillary conjunctivitis (GPC), 89, 94
physical examination of, 91–92
risk factors for, 90
Gleich's syndrome, 73
Global Initiative for Asthma (GINA), 23
Glucagon, in anaphylaxis treatment, 100
Glucocorticoids, 187t
for anaphylaxis, 100

Glucocorticosteroids, in anaphylaxis treatment, 101
Granules, pre-formed, 6
Granulocyte macrophage colony-stimulating factor (GM-CSF), 7, 140
Granulomatosis, bronchocentric, 146

H
Haemophilus influenza, 17
Hapten–carrier complex, 104
Helicobacter pylori, 71
Hepatitis, drug-induced, 107
Hereditary angioedema (HAE), 68, 70, 71
  causes of, 70
  treatment of, 75
Herpes simplex virus (HSV), 83
Hevea brasiliensis, 135
High molecular weight (HMW), 37, 103
High resolution CT (HRCT), 48
Histamine, 6, 61
  H₁ receptor, 6
  H₂ receptor, 6
  H₃ receptor, 6
  H₄ receptor, 6
Honeybees (HBs), 116
  Africanized, 116
Hormonal rhinitis, 12
Hornets, 116
  H₁ receptor, 6
  H₂ receptor, 6
  H₃ receptor, 6
  H₄ receptor, 6
Human leukocyte antigen (HLA), 104
Human papilloma virus (HPV), 83
Humoral immunity, 4
Hygiene hypothesis, 5, 23. *See also* Asthma
Hypereosinophilic syndrome (HES), 140, 142–143, 148
  cardiac involvement of, 143
  neurologic involvement of, 143
  treatment of, 150–151
Hyper IgE syndrome, 165
Hypersensitivity pneumonitis (HP), 40, 44–50
  acute, 46
  causes of, 44
  chronic, 46, 47
  classification of, 44
  definition of, 44
  diagnosis of, 46–49
  differential diagnosis of, 47
  epidemiology of, 44
  etiology of, 44–45, 45t
  outcome of, 49–50

  pathophysiology of, 45–46
  prevention of, 46
  risk factor for, 44
  subacute, 46
  tobacco smoking and, 44
  treatment of, 49
Hypersensitivity reaction, 5t, 61, 85, 96, 103
Hypothyroidism, 12

I
Idiopathic pulmonary fibrosis (IPF), 44
Immotile cilia syndrome, 164
Immune system, 4
  adaptive, 4
  components of, 4
  innate, 4
Immunoglobulin A (IgA), 160
  deficiency, 171
  role of, 4
Immunoglobulin E (IgE), 3, 8, 26, 59
  role of, 4
  types of, 6
  in vitro testing of, 63–64
Immunoglobulin G (IgG), 4
Immunoglobulin range, 191t
Immunotherapy, allergen
  for allergic rhinitis, 14
  clinical efficacy of, 173
  contraindications to, 177–178
  duration of, 173
  failure of, 178
  maintenance doses, 175t
  monitoring of, 178
  outcome of, 179
  pathophysiology of, 173, 174f
  patient education, 178
  perennial aqueous, 194t
  recommended maintenance doses of, 175t
  referral, 178
  side effects and risks of, 177
  treatment of, 173–178
  venom (*see* Venom immunotherapy (VIT))
Indolent systemic mastocytosis (ISM), 157
Infectious fungal sinusitis, 19
Inhaled β₂-agonists, 183t
Inhaled corticosteroids (ICS), 31, 184t.
  See also Steroids
Innate immune system, 4
Insect allergy
  classification of, 117
  diagnosis of, 119–121
  differential diagnosis of, 120
  epidemiology of, 117
  history of, 119

monitoring of, 124
outcomes of, 124
pathophysiology of, 117–118
physical examination of, 119–120
referral, 123t
risk factors for, 118–119
treatment of, 121–123
    for fire ants, 122
    immediate, 121
    venom immunotherapy in, 121–122
Interferon (IFN), 78
Interleukin (IL), 4
Intradermal cutaneous test
    for IgE response measurement, 109
Intradermal skin testing
    for allergy, 60
Intradermal tests, 3
    for food allergy, 131
Intranasal anticholinergics
    for allergic rhinitis treatment, 14
Intranasal antihistamines, 182t
Intranasal corticosteroids, 181t.
        See also Steroids
Intranasal cromolyn
    for allergic rhinitis treatment, 14
Intranasal decongestants, 12
Intranasal steroids
    for allergic rhinitis treatment, 13
Intravenous immunoglobulin (IVIG), 107, 165
In vitro testing, 3
    of IgE, 63–64, 64t
Ipratropium
    for allergic rhinitis treatment, 14
Irritant contact dermatitis (ICD), 85
Isohemagglutinins, saline, 164

K
Keratoconjunctivitis, atopic, 83, 89, 94
Keratoconjunctivitis sicca (KCS), 91
Keratoconus, 83
Kimura's disease, 144

L
Lactate dehydrogenase (LDH), 48
Larva migrans profundus, 143
Latex
    sensitivity, 135
    sensitization, screening questions for, 137t
Latex allergy (LA), 135. See also Latex hypersensitivity
Latex-containing products, 138t
Latex-fruit syndrome, 136
Latex hypersensitivity

clinical presentation of, 136
definition of, 135
diagnostic testing of, 136–137
epidemiology of, 135
pathophysiology of, 135–136
risk factors for, 136
treatment of, 137–138, 137t, 138t
Leukotriene C$_4$ (LTC$_4$), 7
Leukotriene (LT), 7, 9, 89
    modifiers, 31, 74, 185t
Leukotriene receptor antagonists (LTRAs), 32
5-lipoxygenase inhibitor, 32
Lipoxygenase pathway, 7
Local anesthetics (LAs), 113
    classes of, 114t
Löffler's syndrome, 145, 148
    treatment of, 151
Long-acting β_2-agonists (LABAs), 31
Low molecular weight (LMW), 37, 104
    sensitizer, 39
Lung biopsy
    for hypersensitivity pneumonitis diagnosis, 49
Lymphocyte mitogen studies, 191t

M
Macrophage inflammatory protein (MIP), 7
Major basic protein (MBP), 90
Major histocompatibility complexes (MHCs), 104
Mannitol, 56
Mast cell, 6
    activated, 6
    stabilizers, 32
    synthesized cytokines, 7
Mast cell leukemia (MCL), 156
Mastocytosis, 73
    classification of, 155t
    defined, 154
    diagnosis of, 154–157
    outcome of, 158
    pathophysiology of, 154
    treatment of, 157–158
    WHO diagnostic criteria for, 156t
Measles, mumps, and rubella (MMR), 133
Measles, mumps, rubella, and varicella (MMRV), 133
Meibomian gland dysfunction (MGD), 92
Methacholine, 56
Methylprednisolone, 132
Montelukast, for allergic rhinitis, 14
Moraxella catarrhalis, 17
Muckle–Wells syndrome, 73

N

Nasal antihistamines
  for allergic rhinitis treatment, 13
Nasal decongestants
  for allergic rhinitis treatment, 14
Nasal polyps, 11, 12
Nasal provocation testing
  for allergic rhinitis, 13
Nedocromil, in asthma management, 32
Neoprene gloves, usage of, 138
Nitrile gloves, usage of, 138
Nitrogen dioxide exposure and asthma
    risk, 26. *See also* Asthma
Nonallergic rhinitis (NAR), 8
Nonallergic rhinitis with eosinophilia
    syndrome (NARES), 8, 141
Nonsteroidal anti-inflammatory drugs
    (NSAIDs), 10, 26, 106
North American Contact Dermatitis
    Group, 65

O

Occupational asthma (OA)
  agents associated with, 38t
  causes of, 37
  classification of, 37
  definition of, 37
  diagnosis of, 39–42, 41f
  epidemiology of, 37
  irritant-induced, 37, 39
  monitoring of, 42
  outcome of, 42
  pathophysiology of, 37–39
  prevention of, 39
  risk factors for, 39
  sensitizer-induced, 37, 39
  tobacco smoking and, 39
  treatment of, 42
Ocular allergic diseases. *See also specific*
    disorders
  classification of, 89
  clinical presentation of, 90–92
  definition of, 89
  diagnosis for, 90–92
  differential diagnosis of, 92
  epidemiology of, 89
  etiology of, 89
  general treatment of, 92
  medications for, 92–94
  pathophysiology of, 89–90
  referral, 95
  risk factors for, 90
  treatment of, 92, 93t
Ophthalmic antiallergy preparations, 182t
Oral allergy syndrome (OAS), 128

Oral antihistamines
  for allergic rhinitis treatment, 13
Oral corticosteroids. *See also* Steroids
  for allergic rhinitis treatment, 14
Oral decongestants
  for allergic rhinitis treatment, 14
Oral penicillin desensitization, protocol
    for, 111t
Oral sulfonamide desensitization protocol,
    113t
Organic dust toxic syndrome (ODTS), 47
Otitis media, 15
Ouchter-lony double immunodiffusion
    test, 48

P

p-aminobenzoic acid (PABA), 114
Paraphenylenediamine, 86
Patch testing
  in allergic contact dermatitis diagnosis,
    87
  for contact hypersensitivity, 109
  for latex hypersensitivity, 137
Pathogen-associated molecular patterns
    (PAMP), 4
Pattern recognition receptors (PRR), 4
Peak expiratory flow rate (PEFR), 40, 55,
    178
Penicillin (PCN), 104, 112t
  allergy, 111–112
    classification of, 111
    clinical manifestations of, 111
    cross-reactivity of, 112
    desensitization, 112
    epidemiology of, 111
    skin testing for, 112
Peripheral blood lymphocytes
  cell-subset counts of, 192t–193t
Phosphodiesterase inhibitor, 32
p-i concept, 104
Platelet-activating factor (PAF), 7, 154
Pneumococcal polysaccharide vaccination,
    164
Pneumonia
  acute eosinophilic, 144–145
  chronic eosinophilic, 144, 148
Pneumonitis, hypersensitivity, 44–50
  causes of, 44
  classification of, 44
  definition of, 44
  diagnosis of, 46–49
  differential diagnosis of, 47
  epidemiology of, 44
  etiology of, 44–45, 45t
  outcome of, 49–50

pathophysiology of, 45–46
prevention of, 46
risk factor for, 44
tobacco smoking and, 44
treatment of, 49
Pollen-associated FA syndrome, 128
Polyps, nasal, 11
Prausnitz–Kustner test, 62
Prednisone, 132
Pregnancy
and allergic rhinitis, 15
and asthma, 35
Prick skin testing, 60
Primary immunodeficiency diseases, 160.
    See also specific diseases
classification of, 160
common presentations and infectious
    agents, 162t
diagnosis of, 161–171
epidemiology of, 160
history of, 161–163, 161t
immunologic profiles and genetic defects
    of, 166t–170t
physical examination of, 163t
treatment of, 171–172
types and patterns of infection in, 161
workup for
    for suspected combined
        immunodeficiency, 165
    for suspected complement deficiency,
        165
    for suspected phagocyte deficiency,
        165
Priming, 9
Prostaglandin D_2 (PGD$_2$), 7
Prostaglandins, 89
Protein nitrogen unit (PNU), 176
Provocative concentration 20 (PC20), 58
Pseudoallergic reactions, 103
Pseudomonas aeruginosa, 17
Pulmonary disorders and eosinophilia, 144t
Pulmonary eosinophilic granuloma (PEG),
    145–146
Pulmonary function test (PFT), 29, 40,
    48, 51–58, 52t, 53f, 54t, 148
in asthma management, 29
bronchoprovocation testing, 57t
classification of, 51
definition of, 51
diagnosis of, 51–58
and emphysema/chronic obstructive
    pulmonary disease, 55t
flow volume loops, 51
in hypersensitivity pneumonitis
    diagnosis, 48

monitoring of, 51
and restrictive lung disease, 55t
spirometry, 51
Puncture skin testing, 60

R
Rabbit platelet aggregation, 7
Radioallergosorbent test (RAST), 3, 8, 64,
    147
for allergic rhinitis, 12
for food allergy, 131
for insect allergy, 120
Radiocontrast media (RCM), 104
pretreatment protocol for, 110t
Raynaud phenomenon, 107
Reactive airways dysfunction syndrome
    (RADS), 37
Recurrent sinusitis, 17
Reed–Sternberg cells, 143
Regulatory T cells. *See* Tregs
Residual volume (RV), 54
Reverse transcription polymerase chain
    reaction (RT-PCR), 148
Rheumatoid factor (RF), 48
Rhinitis
allergic
    causes of, 8, 9
    definition of, 8
    differential diagnosis of, 11–12, 11t
    perennial, 9
    symptoms of, 8
drug-induced, 12
hormonal, 12
medicamentosa, 12, 15
mixed, 9
nonallergic, 8
vasomotor, 12
Rhinoconjunctivitis, 136
Rhinorrhea, 10
Rhinoscopy, 13
Rhinosinusitis, 15

S
Saccharine test, 20
Saline isohemagglutinins, 164
Samter's triad, 28
Sarcoidosis, 47
Schnitzler's syndrome, 73
Scratch skin test
    for allergy, 62
Seasonal allergic conjunctivitis (SAC), 89
    physical examination of, 91
    risk factors for, 90
Septal deviation, 11
Septal perforation, 11

Serial spirometry, usage of, 40
Serum IgE (sIgE), 117
Serum sickness syndrome, 106. *See also* Drug allergy
Severe combined immunodeficiency (SCID), 80
Short-acting β_2-agonists (SABAs), 30, 31
Shulman's syndrome, 144
Signal transducer and activator of transcription 3 (STAT3), 165
Sinusitis
  acute, 17
  allergic fungal, 19
  biopsy of, 20
  causes of, 17
  ciliary function testing, 20
  classification of, 17
  complications of, 21
  definition of, 16
  diagnosis of
    clinical presentation of, 18
    diagnostic testing, 19–20
    differential diagnosis for, 19, 19t
  epidemiology of, 17
  etiology of, 17
  infectious fungal, 19
  monitoring of, 22
  pathophysiology of, 17–18
  recurrent, 17
  referral of, 21
  rhinoscopy and, 20
  skin prick testing in, 20
  treatment of, 20–21
Skin prick text (SPT), 131
Skin testing
  for allergic rhinitis, 12
  for allergy, 59
  for anaphylaxis, 99
  for atopic dermatitis, 80
  for drug allergy, 112
  for food allergy, 131
  grading system for, 61t
  for insect allergy, 121
  for latex hypersensitivity, 136–137
  for primary immunodeficiency diseases, 165
Solenopsis, 116
Solenopsis invicta, 117
Solitary mastocytoma, 155
Spina Bifida Association of America, 138
Spirometry, 51. *See also* Pulmonary function test (PFT)
  closed-circuit, 52
  criteria for acceptable, 53
  open-circuit, 52

Staphylococcus aureus, 17, 78
Status asthmaticus, 32–33
Stem cell factor (SCF), 154
Steroids
  inhaled, 31, 184t
  intranasal
    for allergic rhinitis, 13
    for sinusitis, 21
  oral
    for allergic rhinitis, 14
    for sinusitis, 21
Stevens-Johnson syndrome (SJS), 107
Styrene gloves, usage of, 138
Sulfonamide allergy, 112–113, 113t
Sweat chloride test, 164
Symblepharon, 91
Systemic lupus erythematosus (SLE), 107
Systemic mastocytosis (SM), 154, 155

T
Tacrolimus, topical, for atopic dermatitis, 81
T-cell–mediated reactions, 103
Telangiectasia eruptive macularis perstans (TEMP), 73
Telangiectasia macularis eruptive perstans (TMEP), 155
T_H1 cells, 4
T_H2 cells, 4
Theophylline, 32
Thrombocytopenia, 108
Thymic stromal lymphopoietin (TSLP), 78
Thyroid-stimulating hormone (TSH), 73
Tobacco smoking
  and hypersensitivity pneumonitis risk, 44
  and occupational asthma, 39
Toll-like receptor (TLR), 160
Total lung capacity (TLC), 54
Toxic epidermal necrolysis (TEN), 107
Toxic oil syndrome, 142
Transforming growth factor (TGF), 4, 154
Transient ischemic attacks (TIAs), 143
Tregs, 4
Trimethoprim-sulfamethoxazole (TMP-SMX), 105
Tropical pulmonary eosinophilia, 145
  treatment of, 151
Tryptase, 6
Tumor necrosis factor (TNF), 6, 46, 154

U
Upper respiratory tract infections (URIs), 161
Urticaria, 2

acute, 69, 73, 128
aquagenic, 72
autoimmune, 69, 73
characteristics of, 70
cholinergic, 72
chronic, 68, 69
classification of, 68
cold, 72
definition of, 68
delayed pressure, 72
diagnosis of, 70–74
differential diagnosis of, 73
epidemiology of, 68–69
etiology of, 69
exercise-induced, 72
outcome of, 75–76
pathophysiology of, 69–70
physical, 72
principles of, 68
solar, 72
treatment of, 74–75
vibratory, 72, 74
Urticaria pigmentosa (UP), 155

V
Vaccination response, 191t
Vasculitis, urticarial, 70, 72

Vasomotor rhinitis, 12
etiology of, 12
Venom immunotherapy (VIT), 120–122
guidelines for, 122t
venom selection in, 121
Vernal keratoconjunctivitis (VKC), 89, 93
physical examination of, 91
risk factors for, 90
Vespidae, 116
Vinyl gloves, usage of, 138
Viral conjunctivitis, 92
Vital capacity (VC), 55
Vocal cord dysfunction (VCD), 28
Volume expansion, for anaphylaxis, 101

W
Wasps, 116
Well's syndrome, 144
White blood cell count and differential
of children, 190t
Wiskott–Aldrich syndrome, 163
World Health Organization (WHO)
diagnostic criteria for mastocytosis, 156t

Y
Yellow jackets (YJs), 116